Live True Publications

Praise for Freedom from IBS:

"Lisa provides a holistic and manageable framework for making any health crisis a hero's journey. Her emphasis on stress reduction and gifting oneself time and space are timeless reminders that we each have the answers unique to ourselves. Lisa's history of IBS hell is a testament that anybody can turn the tides and make peace with their lovely bodies."

~Alisa Elliott Rector, Owner and
CEO of Homegrown Therapy

"...Lisa Thorne…was instrumental in helping me maintain my wellness practices through a difficult time of the pandemic when I was struggling with my own midlife challenges of my business, parenting teenagers, aging parents and mental health and addiction problems of my brother. Her caring and empathetic nature combined with no nonsense and effective coaching strategies are refreshing and impactful, and you can't help but shift your mindset and leave any coaching session with Lisa feeling uplifted and hopeful. On top of being a compassionate and effective coach, she has now shared her story of mastering her own health in The Freedom from IBS book. It is an authoritative insight into not only this syndrome impacting millions of individuals. It provides practical steps to healing combined with her coaching expertise to help people master their mindset and their own health and wellbeing."

~Mindy Gulas, Kinesiologist, Certified
Exercise Physiologist, Lifestyle
Medicine & Wellness Coach

"Lisa Thorne's book is a thoughtful, personal, and empowering exploration of IBS that reflects her own recovery and research, filtered through her experience as a coach. In addition to practical advice for managing symptoms, she offers tools for readers to assess their unique needs and shift their mindset while managing stress. I enjoyed the book's combination of direct experience, a refreshingly wry sense of humor, and a no-nonsense understanding of the impact of digestion, diet, and emotions on IBS symptoms. Her "Freedom Framework" offers clear steps to make the changes that support better health and general well-being for readers struggling with IBS."

~Carol Burbank, Storyweaving

"This disease can be very stigmatizing, but the way [Lisa] has written about it really breaks it down and assists the reader to truly understand the true root of the cause of the problem. This is a great read and you will greatly benefit by investing your time reading this book to learn how to be on the healing road to wellness."

~D. VanderMeer, Licensed Massage Therapist

Find Freedom from IBS:
A Holistic Approach to Wellness, Gut Health, and Getting Your Life Back

2nd Edition

Lisa Thorne

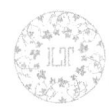

Live True Publications

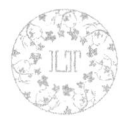

Live True Publications
PO Box 966
Coloma, MI 49038

Copyright © 2023 by Lisa Thorne

All rights reserved.

No part of this publication may be reproduced, distributed, or transmitted in any form or by any means, including photocopying, recording, or other electronic or mechanical methods, without the prior written permission of the publisher, except in the case of brief quotations embodied in critical reviews and certain other noncommercial uses permitted by copyright law. For permission requests, write to the publisher at the address below.

ISBN: 979-8-9879844-0-6

Published by Live True Publications
This book is the second edition of Live True Publication's Freedom from IBS, dedicated to publishing books that support wellness, choice, and joy.

Dedication

I dedicate this book to every one of you
desiring to make long-lasting positive change,
and having the diligence, determination,
and courage to take action.

DISCLAIMER

This book is not intended as a substitute for the medical advice of physicians. The reader should regularly consult a physician in matters relating to his/her health and particularly with respect to any symptoms that may require diagnosis or medical attention. The purpose of this book is to convey information.

It should not be interpreted as medical advice, and is not intended to diagnose, treat, or cure your condition, or to be a substitute for advice from your physician or other healthcare professional. The methods discussed in this program are intended to support health and healing, not to replace medical treatment.

Whether you choose conventional treatments, alternative treatments, or both, it is imperative that you work closely with a doctor or healthcare professional to properly diagnose and treat your condition, and to monitor your progress.

CONTENTS

Pick Your Battles

Introduction

Never in my wildest dreams (or nightmares) would I have thought I would write a book about such an indelicate topic as my digestion.

It has taken a lot of practice to be able to talk about my symptoms, the primary one being a horrific and endless case of "the trots". Rest assured, this book is not only about poo per se, but (without creating unnecessary visuals), it does rear its ugly head. Coping with Number Two is a major component of what makes living with this functional disorder sometimes tremendously difficult, but is only part of the diminished quality of life.

As anyone with IBS knows, the negative effects are *far more* **than just the end result (everything sounds like a pun, doesn't it)**. Far from being all in our head, as well-meaning friends, family, and coworkers may suggest, IBS can be debilitating to the point of serious depression. I now believe that I have at different times experienced a wide range of IBS symptoms, literally from head to foot, and in widely varying degrees, possibly since I was an adolescent. It took me years to understand that what I experienced with my digestive adventures wasn't normal, and to slowly try to rule out food allergies, or food intolerances (there's a difference), or other "actual" diseases that have similar symptoms to IBS, like colitis, or celiac, or Crohn's, or colon cancer.

I've spent lots of money on varying modalities, lots of time on my own research, and lots of energy searching for a practitioner that would "solve" my problems and not just send me down yet another rabbit hole. I've learned quite a few things along the way, and while my experience is probably not exactly the same as another's, I have found what works based on the thousands of hours of research and testing and experimenting and documenting and reading and living I have done with this disorder. I hope to save you some of the agony you might endure without some of this information, and **hope to help empower you to forge your own path to wellness**, just as I have done. I am now what I consider to be free of the symptoms of IBS, and have been for several years. My strongest desire is that you can get there too.

While you may be hoping I dole out lists of exactly what you can eat or what you cannot (as I would have been hoping for too, just a few years ago), the keys to my recovery are found within four key areas, only one of them related to what I put into my mouth as food. It was only when I zoomed out to the big picture of my overall health and wellbeing that I really started to see results.

The first major step was a critical shift in my mindset. I know this is such a buzzword, a very trendy concept, but it was pivotal in a very real way, in allowing me the ability to seek answers beyond those I had been reaching for, because I finally reached a point where I would accept nothing else than getting better.

Our health is impacted in either positive or negative ways by so many factors, most of them decisions and choices we make to either support health, or, conversely, "power through," or even insist we do not have choices. *Wellness is much more than what we eat, or how much exercise we get. It is greatly impacted by our frame of mind, our emotional health, and our kindness to ourselves.* Yes, there were factors directly related to the food choices I made, but the overall incredible recovery I achieved was due to all of these factors, as a whole.

What's interesting to me is that I had improved nearly every other area of my life thanks to critical shifts in my mindset, being attentive to my emotional wellbeing, and recognizing and employing healthy choices. The last thing to improve I hadn't realized was within my control: my physical health related to IBS. I felt like a victim and worse, like I had absolutely no choice in the state of my digestive system.

It was only when I melded my healing journey into one holistic approach, instead of focusing only on food, that I very quickly found relief.

Letting Go of What You Know

For you to fully absorb the information I share here, I invite you to do something that may at first feel counterintuitive, even scary: *I ask you to forget all that you think you know about your journey with your symptoms and suffering thus far.* Forget, or at least allow, that what you have identified as the culprit, or perhaps several culprits, (you know, the foods that seem to have almost no rhyme or reason as to why they might causing issues, which leave you constantly wondering if the next food may also throw you into a tailspin), and just be open to a new way of categorizing not only what you eat, but how you are eating it. There is a concept in Buddhism of cultivating a "beginner's mind", and though I will not be suggesting primarily or even any Buddhist practices, I do encourage you to be open, attempt an attitude of eagerness and possibility, to what I share with you here.

We may have a tendency to say "I've tried that, it doesn't work" about a myriad of different occasions in our lives, and dismiss that which is being proposed before it even has a chance to make its case. But the reality, in a lot of cases, is that we did try it…but maybe only once, or maybe not under the same conditions, or maybe not without considering numerous other factors, or maybe all of the above. Look at this way: *if all the limitations you may currently believe you must live under to operate in the world with your IBS symptoms could be simplified, even eliminated, wouldn't that be worth trying again?*

I welcome you to set aside the preconceptions you may have, and allow this information to just soak into your inner knowing. See if it feels right. If some of it doesn't, there may be other pieces of information that ring true, but even so, you are no worse for considering these options. And, if some things do sit right with you, it does begin to make sense and show you a new way, a way that is manageable and makes sense, and seems to improve your symptoms, well, that's a lovely possibility, isn't it?

You can, and I mean no pun whatsoever, trust your gut. If something you read really resonates, listen to your inner knowing. Trust that your body, your self, your knowledge and all the things that only you know about yourself, may be telling you. Take with you from this book what resonates, and just leave the rest. You can always come back to this book. It will be here for you. You may find things that help you today, and later in your journey, you find things that help you then. *This is our journey in life.*

The Freedom Framework

I coach from a framework of three basic principles that so far seem to hold true for any event, situation, or desire we have in our lives. I have come to call it the Freedom Framework, because following it is so freeing, so liberating, especially when compared to the knots we can tie ourselves in trying to follow someone else's plan or diet, or berating ourselves for not doing something we said we would, or for thinking a disingenuous thought about someone we love (or ourselves).

As a general rule, it is much easier to allow, versus push against, to be forgiving of our choices instead of speaking harshly in our minds, to be kinder, just a little bit kinder, as we navigate the many paths each day brings us.

And the more I did that - tried a little kinder thought, a little less resistant path, a little more allowing decision - the easier and better and kinder and happier each moment seemed to get. You may be thinking this doesn't have a thing to do with your current digestive hell, but I assure you, it has *everything* to do with it.

The three main points of the Freedom Framework are:

1. **Striving for the next better thing [emotion, food, thought, experience, relationship, job, choice, decision]. Always.** *You are just looking to better your experience, based on how you feel in the moment, so that every choice becomes better and more fulfilling and more true to what you desire, in that moment in time, based on what you know to be true.* Each moment you collect more information, and each moment gives you another opportunity to cultivate a slightly better, slightly more informed, slightly kinder and slightly more enjoyable experience. Keeping this point of reference, this point of focus if you will, can really fuel your momentum to get through things you may have perceived as difficult, because you are so aware that there is so much to gain. *Then, it suddenly seems the hard things become easier!*

2. Embracing what is unique to YOU, and understanding WHY. **What is right for the masses is not necessarily right for the individual.** Generalizations and information help guide you, but ultimately, the specifics of what you as an individual need based on your own unique wellness journey is what you must base your decisions upon. **Despite what it may sometimes feel like, Google does not know you as well as you know yourself.** *Coming to trust that you are making the right decisions despite "evidence" to the contrary is an important and significant part of embracing your ability to be well and make wonderful choices for your own continued well being.*

**Knowing that something is right or is not right for you
also helps you advocate on your own behalf, and to
stand in sureness of what you need for balance (and
ultimately, to feel good).**

3. Mastering continued growth! Or, I could phrase this as,
    **understanding what is right for you in the moment will
    inevitably change as you continue to evolve, and as life
    continues to shift!** We are all different and unique
    individuals, and we ourselves continue to change, evolve,
    grow, become older, become healthier, become ill,
    experience moments of joy, moments of relaxation and
    busy-ness and anger and frustration and so on. And,
    therefore, our needs change moment by moment too. Your
    diet, for example, need not reflect each and every
    undulation of your physical reality or emotional world, but
    you do sometimes need different things based on where
    you are in your life, and learning to trust that, though you
    may be choosing differently than your norm, what you are
    choosing is right for you in the moment is key to the
    freedom and health you are ultimately seeking.

The Freedom Framework not only applies to your relationship with
your decisions around food and your physical health, it applies to
and works with relationships to others, with self-care, with every
choice you have to make and with every thought you think, to
bring you to a better, happier, easier, healthier existence. It works
because you will grow to understand:

*   Intuitively what the next best choice is for you
*   Why it is the best choice in the moment for you

7

- *That there is no failure, no going backward, no keeping score, no guilt, and no shame*
- **What is best for you specifically; not for "everyone" or "most people", but for YOU**
- That life happens (conflict, hardship, curveballs, travel, sickness, happy events, hard events, boring events), and you will be ready and armed with the knowledge of how to proceed with health, ease, and happiness

I lay out this Freedom Framework here at the beginning of this book, in hopes of encouraging you to just allow the information to sink into your realm of possibilities.

As you consume the words on these pages, trust that if something sounds easy or at least easier than what you've been doing (Framework #1), that's a good indication it may be a good thing to try for yourself (Framework #2). And, as you continue to try new approaches, trust that your approaches will likely change (Framework #3) as you heal and learn. Expecting change is a lovely way to not be thrown out of whack when things do shift. Change is a good thing! We can learn to eagerly anticipate things out of our norm, and as we obtain more knowledge and understanding, we become better and better equipped to deal with anything that comes our way.

A Tale of Woe: My Story

My "tummy troubles" started as an adolescent. I can recall such severe cramps that I would break out in a sweat. I did not know it was abnormal, until a friend saw me in the backseat of a car, holding my breath and bracing my body in such a way that she must have recognized. She said, "My sister gets those too". The cramps evolved over the next decades into a variety of other symptoms, but I think ultimately those pangs were related to the very beginning of what I now consider my journey with IBS.

Fast-forward several decades, and many years of increasingly problematic symptoms that were so constant in my life, I was oddly not even fully aware of my slow decline. **It crept up on me to the point that I didn't even realize I was living my life based completely on the possibility that my digestion would not cooperate.** I was accepting (or, often not) invitations to events, with my very first thought always one of where or if there would be a bathroom available, and what I would do for food if it was an event that involved eating, because eating meant I would likely need a bathroom, pronto. Mornings were so consistently terrible for me, that if the event was in the morning, it was a definite no, except for those things I absolutely had to do, like go to class and then in later years, go to a job.

Only when it finally dawned on me that I was living my life around my possible digestive reaction and being bound tighter and tighter by the restrictions of what I thought I could tolerate, that *I became desperate for a solution.* I had experienced a pretty steady decline in wellness in terms of anything resembling normal digestion, when I hit such a low, I became desperate to find something that worked, something to help me live my life again. My relationships were suffering. My emotions were a mess. My stress was through the roof. There was sometimes just horrific pain. I had almost given up on the medical (both traditional and alternative) world being able to do anything for me, when test after test revealed "nothing was wrong", and well-meaning practitioners suggested one or two things that ultimately seemed to – once again – help for a little while, and then plummet me back down, sometimes worse than before.

I just could not seem to find anything to help. All my years prior to this point had been at least tolerable, but I eventually reached a stage of desperation. I was eating an extremely limited diet, even by restricted dieting standards, and was still in a state of extreme discomfort every morning, and often into the day, a "flare" that lasted literally about three years.

If you're not familiar with the term "flare up", it can mean any number of things depending on who the person is and what their symptoms are, but the commonality between them is that the digestive process is so out of control as to be unpredictable and to wreak havoc with the ability to live your life in any normal way.

I combed, as I had been doing, the internet for anything, any information that could help, when I found what I thought was a gold-mine. A particular fiber supplement was being marketed as the cure for IBS. I mean, it was specifically for IBS, so it had to work, right?! I had already tried fiber supplements, multiple kinds - guess what? They never helped for long, and some made it even worse, but since this one was specific to IBS, I ordered it, and as I waited the handful of days for the delivery, my hopes soared that it would be the answer to my prayers. When it arrived, I quickly opened the package, and read the instructions to add the supplement in powder form to each meal.

Hope is a funny thing, isn't it? After all the attempts in the past, all the times I'd tried something new and gotten burned, all the times I'd had my hopes dashed, yet I still went full-throttle with this supplement. Guess what? This time, the supplement marketed for solving my IBS symptoms absolutely wrecked me.

The first day I used it, my symptoms changed so much that I thought it must have been helping, even though I wouldn't have described the changes as necessarily positive - just different. The next day, I had alarming pain, was passing mucus, and by the second evening, was passing blood and what looked like tissue. My god. How?! How could this have happened, when this product was marketed to people with sensitive intestines?!

I wrote an email to the owner of the company, and explained what was happening. She assured me that there was "no possible way" the supplement could hurt me, but then she said, "Be sure to introduce it slowly, starting with about a ¼ teaspoon per meal." I was stunned, and upset, and scared, because what I had done was add the entire little packet, which looked like a little single-serve packet (like a sugar packet, only fiber) to each meal, which was about 2 tablespoons worth. That's about 12 times the amount she recommended I begin with. I was much too scared to even be upset with her, or with the company for not making it more clear (like abundantly clear!) to start slowly.

I was upset with myself for not being more careful, for trusting. I was terrified because my body, my poor intestines, really seemed to be injured from this, despite her assurances that the fiber could not possibly cause any harm. Well, it had. It not only caused harm, it caused me to have the worst flare up of my entire life, escalating my three-year long flare into a state of pain, physical evidence of damage, and terror . The event really spiraled me down into true fear that I had done something terrible to my body.

As happens in life, this mistake with the supplement quantity turned out to be a huge blessing, because ultimately, it helped finally figure out what worked for me. It forced me to hit rock bottom as they say, and to finally say, "Enough!". It, strangely, empowered me to seek my own truths, quit relying on what others (well-meaning or not) said or promised or suggested. I figured out how to turn the tide of my health, and now, years later, it's still working. **I have only gotten better and better, and better.**

I consider myself now to be **living IBS free**. I can eat *more variety* of foods than I have in decades, with few to no side effects. This doesn't mean I make poor food choices - on the contrary, if you think you can get to a point where you just eat anything with no concern for smart, healthy choices, think again. *Nobody - and I mean nobody - can live long without repercussions from* *unhealthy food choices.* I do mean I don't have to analyze every meal, I don't have to look up menus ahead of going to a restaurant to plot out what is "safe" or "hopefully safe" for me to eat, I don't have to order specialty preparations ("no gluten", "no bun", "no cheese" etc.), unless I want them. I can choose very easily and quickly what is the best choice for me, because I now understand exactly what works.

I am excited to share what I've learned with you, in hopes of helping you, and the millions of other people struggling as I was. **I make no claims to "curing" your symptoms. You have to do that, and I'll give you tons of information to help you get there.** There is no magic solution here. There's not a certain pill, or a specific diet, so if you're looking for something that will let you just keep eating whatever you want and living however you want, this is not the right information for you. The path to the incredible wellness I now have was a journey, a process, and I believe I have pinpointed the critical areas needed to turn the dial on wellness. **I have gained a great understanding of what works, and why.** *Your journey can look however you choose, and my hope is that you will gain the insights and information that help you shape the fastest possible path to health and freedom from your symptoms.*

I understand if you want to skip these beginning chapters, and head straight to the "how I did it" and "what worked for me" parts. Before you do that, let me assure you that it is not just what you eat that is causing your symptoms. There are many other factors to consider, and just changing your diet without addressing the other areas will lead you where I ended up - so desperate to find a solution but living each day as if there wasn't one. I am a holistic wellness coach, and even I missed how significant the big picture was in the throes of my illness. **The fastest and most long lasting method for you to achieve wellness is to recognize that *all the parts contribute to the whole*.** And that starts with how you think about your symptoms, and your possibilities for wellness.

The Story You Tell

Changing your mindset around your illness is key to being able to move toward healing. **It is not only how your symptoms and subsequent needs impact others, or how you feel about your symptoms and needs, but also about the simple concept of whether or not you actually believe you can get well.**

Do you believe that you are doomed to a life of increasingly difficult symptoms, or that you will "never" heal, as so much of the literature out there suggests? I believed it too. Then came the day, after running late each morning for days in a row, because I simply could not get away from a bathroom longer than 15 minutes without having to run back in, after having such anxiety my hands visibly shook on a regular basis, and I couldn't get a night's rest without waking multiple times to literally run to the bathroom, when **I finally said to myself, "I'm not living like this anymore. This cannot go on." I became determined to find my way out. And I did.**

One of the greatest gifts you can give yourself is permission to rewrite your story, to define yourself in ways that feel better, seem more true, and allow you freedom and flexibility. "But wait - what the heck is she even talking about?!", you may be thinking. "I thought this was a book about finding freedom from IBS! **What does 'my personal narrative' have to do with my digestion?!"** *The truth is, so very many of the patterns we follow in our day-to-day choices have to do with the beliefs we have about ourselves, and are related to the stories we tell about ourselves.*

Here's an example you may be able to relate to: I have a 20-year-old client whose family regularly complained about her food limitations. She explained to them that she just wasn't able to eat certain foods, and though they love her and care for her, they couldn't understand such limitations. They saw her needs to have alternative food options as deprivation for her, and hardship for them to accommodate.

My young client found herself, sadly but understandably, not wanting to associate with her family, who she loved greatly, and worse, sometimes just eating whatever they served rather than drawing unwanted attention to her needs, which resulted in pain and flare ups. Along with the despair that accompanies the unpredictability of IBS is often shame or embarrassment about causing problems, or being a hindrance or even nuisance for others.

Some sufferers feel that they are being needy, or that others resent their limitations. These beliefs come from stories that we are either taught about being polite, not focusing on our own needs, and not inconveniencing others, or stories we tell ourselves along the same lines, of believing we aren't worth troubling over, and that others are unduly burdened by our needs. When you can revise those stories to allow you to care for yourself, and insist upon your needs, a lot of the mental anguish can be resolved.

After some sessions together, my client came to realize her IBS is not really different from having a broken leg - it's not her fault, it's an inconvenience for her as well as sometimes for others; she didn't ask for it nor does she like it; and, she sometimes needs accommodating to help her be comfortable in different places (venues, experiences, atmospheres, activities). When she shared this frame of a broken leg analogy with her family, they realized they weren't honoring her needs. They were ultimately able to see her limitations and challenges in an empathetic way, and were much more able to want to help and accommodate her. Her mother even eventually shared that she too, experienced digestive issues, but had never felt she could trouble anyone about it.

If you have "accepted" that your IBS is here to stay, you are not alone. Many hundreds of thousands, if not millions, of others buy into this wide-spread notion, for the simple reason that it is written in all kinds of literature, that our medical providers say it to us, that the Facebook groups and self-help books all support and condone this very limiting belief. This is the first of several items in this book that will go against the grain of common knowledge, but with good reason. I have found complete freedom from IBS. It is as if I not only never had it, but I feel better than I have in decades. **It is absolutely possible to find freedom from your symptoms, but not if you don't believe it.**

Let me share a truth with you: **You are NOT your diagnosis. You are NOT your symptoms. Sit with that for a minute. Whisper it to yourself, and let that truth wash over you.**

Perhaps you say:

> "I will never get well"
> "No matter what I do, I can't seem to get better"
> "I have tried everything" "I tried that; it doesn't work"
> "I can't ever eat that [very specific food that you avoid in all forms]"

Any of these statements *could* be true, but I want to encourage you to first recognize the limitations these beliefs are creating for you, and secondly, to be open to the possibility that what you suspect is causing or is the state of your symptoms, may not be exactly what you think.

Consider, "I will never get well." There is something to be said for being brave and accepting the fate of our paths, but there is also something to be said for being pulled into a story that keeps you from thriving. If you really believed you could never get well, why are you here?

I'll tell you why. Because you WANT to get well, and therein lies the dichotomy. **You have a desire to be free of the agony and unknowns of life with symptoms of IBS, and yet, you don't believe you can be.** It's possible this is causing you to be mentally stuck in a rut of wanting something that you tell yourself isn't possible to have. What a terrible place to be! I know this from my own experience. I see similar narratives with many of my coaching clients, related to not only their health, but also their relationships, their careers, their spiritual journeys, and more. The common refrain is "I just feel stuck" It is nearly immobilizing. I can hear you already saying, "But there are people all over the world who have something wrong with them that won't heal, and who want something different!" That's true - and this is true for them as well: *Changing the way you frame the situation can make every difference for how you heal and how you improve your situation.*

"I will never get well" can shift to a slightly more positive, less absolute statement of "I would like to get well" or "I would like to feel better", which can then become "I would like to know how to feel better" and "I would really like to understand what I can do to feel good" and so forth. When you pair the desire of desperately wanting to get better with the opposing belief that you never will, how could you possibly make progress? But when you shift to a more empowering statement of desiring to feel better, of seeking information that helps you feel better, you allow for these things to come into your existence. It is a subtle yet significant shift.

Allowing a New Version

Since the antagonist of our story, poo, must sometimes be discussed, I must take a moment to thank Microsoft Word's synonym function which offered peep, toot, bleep, and beep-beep as alternatives to the word, poop.

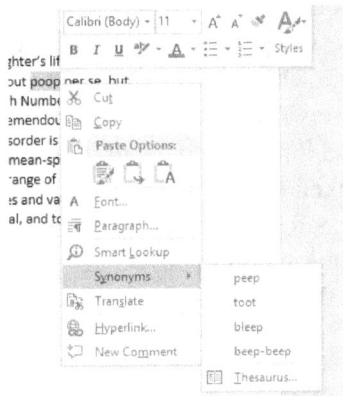

I hope it makes you laugh, because your sense of humor is a huge factor in regaining your health and adjusting your frame of mind. Not only your digestive health, but your health over all benefits from letting go, not taking things too seriously, letting things be easy and light. I know, easier said than done – I really do know!

I know that when you are tied to a bathroom or experience extreme anxiety at the thought of venturing farther than walking distance from a toilet, or when you wake abruptly in the night because you've got to use the bathroom NOW, it's very hard to "lighten up". I understand, and I've found a few tricks that have helped me tremendously.

And I promise, I am not going to tell you to "just meditate"! Although I think that meditating is wonderful and life-improving, and health-improving and soul- and spirit-improving, I have historically found it really difficult to meditate, particularly when in the throes of a flare up or when experiencing high stress or agitation; often I felt I didn't have the time, or if I "made" time (squeezing it in between papers or jobs or errands or chores or whatever else life as a single working-multiple-jobs parent and taking college courses had on my to-do list), my mind was in such a whirl of all the things I wasn't doing that I didn't benefit a lot from the meditation. (Yes, I do realize the irony in that.) But hey, it just didn't work well for me for a long time, and instead I eventually found other ways to calm my soul and lift my spirit and lighten up. I can now meditate "effectively" and I do so, often, with joy and ease. I find it remarkably calming and energizing at the same time. It's taken me a long time to get to truly being present. If meditating works for you, that's great, and keep it up! Go for it, I say, if meditation is calling you. If not, or in addition, you might try a few of these things.

The worst thing to say to someone who is feeling stressed is to "calm down" or "relax". *But ya gotta.* I mean this in the kindest, most supportive way. We can get so tangled in our net of misery that the most beautiful moments can pass us by without us finding even an iota of relief from them. If that's the case, where life feels so heavy and you are resistant to the joy if only because it feels so risky to feel "good," because you know you'll just feel awful again in a skinny minute, then it's all the more important to allow those good feelings. Be brave, and just let them wash over you. Seek them out, wherever you can.

Even if you find you are watching from a distance, as an enjoyable event occurs in your life, but you don't feel fully present or able to even smile inside, if you're just uber focused on the symptoms crashing through you or so terrified of the symptoms about to rage, finding ways to distract yourself from this hell becomes tremendously helpful. It eases the stress response, even for just a moment, and your body gets a split second of respite.

Holding, holding, holding that stress, fear, anxiety, tension at a constant is a tough cycle to break from, but doing so makes room for a little more releasing, a smidge more relaxation, a touch of calm, a glimpse of serenity, and even a little light, a little desire for levity, for some ease, some relief from the doom and darkness.

Remember I said I didn't take well to meditation at all, but now I meditate and even enjoy it? It's only because I was able to let a little lightness in that I was able to get to a larger experience of letting go. **It's about baby steps.** Here is a nice steady pace you can take to introduce more ease into your days:

Find ways to laugh. Hang out with funny people. If you don't have funny people in your life, find some! Subscribe to the Comedy channel. Turn straight to the Funny Pages of the newspaper or magazines you read. Follow comedians you like on Twitter. Pay attention to what people really say – most of it is hilarious if you really listen (even if they don't mean it that way)! Levity is significant. *The power of being able to laugh, to find the lighter, more playful version of any situation is key to your freedom (not just with IBS).*

Likewise, be attentive to what brings you down. Is there a particular person who you dread being around? Then remove yourself from interaction with them. You have control of your choices! If you are saying, "But I have to work with the dweeb!", note that I said "remove from interaction" - this does not have to happen physically. You can still be physically present, but you can shift your presence to a place of observation, or spectator, watching the person's behavior and banter as if on a screen.

You can distance yourself from stressful people and situations by simply observing. Becoming curious about why they may do or say what they do, without passing judgment. You are a detective. Just collecting information, watching, quietly observing. You will likely notice things about the person that let you not only distance yourself from the stress you had been feeling, but also to see the person in a different light. I am not going to suggest you will find great compassion and become fast friends, but I will say that their behavior may not have the significant impact upon you it did before you practiced this. Practice is key. We think of someone or something that is stressful, that we desperately want to find more ease with or escape from, and we try to observe. It works for a split second, the first time, and then we fall into response mode, of interacting again, or being upset about the situation. Practice! Try again! The next time, we last a bit longer, we gain a better foothold. Practice. *Everything we wish to do to better ourselves and our life experience requires practice at first.* Could you tie your shoes the first time you tried? Was it hard? Did you practice until you got it? How about now? How is that shoe-tying experience? A no-brainer, right? So, was it worth it?

There are lots of stressful things happening on the global stage, and even in our own backyards. I sincerely give you permission to stop watching the news if it makes you sad, angry, frustrated, or upset. *When you're experiencing such a volatile and draining syndrome as IBS, you must gather your forces around you and conserve your energies for healing.* I promise you, once you have regained your health, the news reels you thought you couldn't live without will still be there for you, ready and waiting. Your civic duty as a news-consumer is not going to make the world crumble if you step back. If the world stage is bringing you down, but you find you cannot live without the news, or you cannot live with yourself without consuming the news, at the very least equal it out with intentional consumption of things light, things of beauty, things that bring joy or at least make you smile, even for a moment.

Join Facebook groups that regularly share funny or lovely things – I don't mean mean-spirited political rants that make you feel venomous or vengeful; but actual funny, actually beautiful, beautifully kind, things. Go to Facebook or Instagram, type in Comedy in the search bar, and a bunch of options will pop up! Type in Sacred Geometry and tap into the beauty and magic of the world. Search for Amazing Animals. Type in Amazing World. Find groups that share things about elephants, or octopi. When you like, follow, or join, magically your feed will include posts that bring you levity, joy, and often a bit of what feels like magic.

Set a goal to find things that really get you going – belly laughs, tears rolling down the cheeks with laughter, things that make you chuckle again later when you recall them. **This is a really big deal!** *IBS can get you so wrapped up in the anxiety, the awfulness, that learning to let go and let life be enjoyable, even for a just a moment is really important and so good for your health and your spirit.*

Find humorous ways to describe your experiences. **How we talk about our experience with IBS is as important as the thoughts we think about it.** When we describe our experiences in desperation and despair, we don't leave room for levity or moving forward. It mires us down in the hardship of it; we want to be able to keep moving forward despite the muck. **Humor is much like placing wide planks over a muddy path to give us something to balance upon.** *We feel lighter, less stuck.*

The point of course is to try to balance out some of the misery, and while you might think this book is, itself, so far full of *peep* and though you might be ready to toss it, please don't underestimate the importance of the power of perception. *When we focus on the wretchedness of the experience that is IBS, we will ultimately see and experience only more wretchedness.*

My experience with IBS is one of a very cyclical nature, a bit of a chicken or the egg scenario, where I often considered whether the anxiety (worry over a possible flare up) caused the symptom, or if the symptom (a very real flare) caused the anxiety. What I have found is that both are true, and once I finally figured out what worked for me, through what ultimately became the handful of months of my rapid recovery (yes, several months felt rapid after grappling with these chains for decades), the anxiety was one of the longest lasting symptoms and the hardest to finally release. It is still the first sign that reappears when anything questionable is happening with my digestive system. Perhaps I have trust issues (okay, I do have trust issues; that's another book), but nevertheless the fear of *an episode* to put it delicately lingered well into the days and then weeks where there was no episode at all…learning to trust and let go of the worry was the ultimate success. I am mostly, as in 99% of my waking hours, free of worrying about peep, toot, bleep, and yes, even beep-beep. And I firmly believe you can be too.

Perception is, as I alluded earlier, a big player in this game we call IBS. It is, in fact, a superjock in the game we call Life. *What we focus on, we find and how we perceive the experiences in our lives shapes our meaning of them.* We may ascribe to an event meanings and emotions of fear, anxiety, or misery, or alternatively, we might choose to assign humor, lessons learned, and useful information to the very same event. It is within our control. The stories we tell are important, and how we phrase things is critically important. Empowering ourselves with speech like "I will succeed, I will get well, I am finding what works, I am healing" versus "I never, I won't, I can't, etc." make an enormous difference. If you think it's silly, or if you think it can't possibly make a difference, I challenge you to just try it. I think you'll find that not only do you not feel worse, or create more symptoms, but you will find that you will open to new and different possibilities you hadn't seen or considered before, like a flower blooming in the sun.

Understanding What is Important

Very briefly, let's define some of the words and phrases I use in this book. There will be no quiz.

Vocabulary

Anxiety: "Apprehensive uneasiness or nervousness usually over an impending or anticipated ill" and "an abnormal and overwhelming sense of apprehension and fear often marked by physical signs (such as tension, sweating, and increased pulse rate)..."[1] I use anxiety and stress sometimes interchangeably, only because they seemed to always go hand in hand. *My anxiety stressed me out.* **When I was stressed, I became anxious that I would have a flare up. You get the picture.**

Diarrhea: Loose stool. It does not have to be "watery", like with the flu. It can simply by non-formed stool. It can be unformed with some formed pieces, it can be watery and/or unformed. The key is that it is likely urgent as well.

Digestion: "The process of making food absorbable by mechanically and enzymatically breaking it down into simpler chemical compounds in the digestive tract"[2] You probably knew this, but it's helpful to remember that our ability to digest food is key to our physical health and that the process is a fairly simple, basic function.

Flare/Flare up: I use this to describe a digestive event that takes over your world, for a period of time. One urgent trip to the

---

[1] https://www.merriam-webster.com/dictionary/anxiety
[2] https://www.merriam-webster.com/dictionary/digestion

bathroom is not necessarily a flare up, but several, or many, could be. Having discomfort at every meal, or just after every meal, could also be considered a flare-up. If you tend to be on the constipated side of IBS, your flare-ups may be the frustrating pain, gas, and bloating associated with not being able to go. You likely know what you consider a flare up for you, and it may not look the same as mine, or Jane's or Bill's or Enrique's. It's okay that they don't look the same. You identify your flare-ups however you need to so that you can identify when you are having them less and less frequently.

Gastrocolic reflex: "[I]s one of a number of physiological reflexes controlling the motility, or peristalsis, of the gastrointestinal tract. It involves an increase in motility of the colon in response to stretch in the stomach and byproducts of digestion in the small intestine. The small intestine also shows a similar motility response"[3]. We will talk more about this in the next section.

Homeostasis: "a relatively stable state of equilibrium or a tendency toward such a state between the different but interdependent elements or groups of elements of an organism, population, or group"[4]. In this case we are talking about the body's wonderful and strong desire to find balance.

IBS-D: Irritable Bowel Syndrome, predominantly presenting with diarrhea

IBS-C: Irritable Bowel Syndrome, predominantly presenting with constipation

IBS-M: Irritable Bowel Syndrome, presenting with both diarrhea and constipation, like a pendulum swinging

---

[3] https://www.wikidoc.org/index.php/Gastrocolic_reflex
[4] https://www.merriam-webster.com/dictionary/homeostasis

Motility: "The ability of the muscles of the digestive tract to undergo contraction"[5] Again, in this sense, contraction is good, and we like that our intestines can contract, to help peristalsis along.

Peristalsis: "Successive waves of involuntary contraction passing along the walls of a hollow muscular structure (such as the esophagus or intestine) and forcing the contents onward"[6] Though it may not sound like it, peristalsis is a good thing - trust me when I say we like it when our intestines do their involuntary contractions. Our goal is to help them do it in a way that is manageable.

Run to the bathroom/be preoccupied with the bathroom/tied to a toilet: This probably doesn't have to be defined, but for the sake of eliminating (a-hem) any questions, here I mean that you either have an urgent need to evacuate your bowels, likely due to diarrhea, and possibly on a repeated basis, or you are unable to go, and therefor spending a lot of time trying.

Stress: "A state resulting from stress, especially one of bodily or mental tension resulting from factors that tend to alter an existent equilibrium"[7] This definition is pretty spot on, but let me also add, just because your everyday life is full of demanding circumstances doesn't mean it's not also stressful. *It is very possible that your life, day after day, is a point of stress.* Telling yourself that "it's always been this way" or that "I've never had trouble with my demanding life before" isn't an accurate way of looking at or managing the stress in your life. **Just because it's "always" been there does NOT mean it hasn't been quietly impacting you! Experiencing stress over long periods of time will, eventually, inevitably, have an impact.**

Trusted Health Practitioner: I say this instead of saying "your doctor" because you may choose to use a medical doctor (MD) for

---

[5] https://www.merriam-webster.com/dictionary/motility
[6] https://www.merriam-webster.com/dictionary/peristalsis
[7] https://www.merriam-webster.com/dictionary/stress

your care, or a nurse practitioner (NP), or a physician's assistant (PA), or a naturopath (ND), or an osteopath (OD), or a massage therapist, a chiropractor, a dietician, an acupuncturist, or anyone you trust who is an expert in whatever it is you are going to them for. The key word in this is Trusted. *You must have confidence with your health practitioners, and you must feel safe in voicing your desires.*

Urgency: A sudden need to use the bathroom, typically due to diarrhea.

Wellness team: People in your life you look to for guidance, knowledge, support, and care. This can include your trusted health practitioners (there may be many, there may be only one), family or friends, and anyone who you can lean on and who "gets it."

The Body's Relationship with Digestion

A very key thing to understand about digestion, and about our bodies in general, is that it's *always* striving for balance. Although it may seem to swing from one extreme to another, the body is looking for what is called *homeostasis,* and **just as with a pendulum swinging, *it must sometimes go wide before settling back into a normal range.*** Sometimes, that pendulum swings longer than we think it should or want it to. There are of course options to arrest the moment, such as antidiarrheals or laxatives depending on which way you're swinging, but just as grabbing a pendulum to halt it is rather abrupt, so too can be the use of over-the-counter or prescribed interrupters. The trick is to use them in a way that is more gentle, much like if you were trying to slow the blade of a ceiling fan without hurting your hand. Thinking of how to be gentle with your body, your digestive system, is a really good approach to helping your body heal and find that balance it wants just as badly as you do. Your body really does seek balance, and it really is trying to get everything working ship shape..

If you are feeling like, "Oh my gosh, sometimes it seems like this [food] helps and sometimes it seems like it hurts," it's probably true. Sometimes you may tolerate certain foods and sometimes you may not tolerate the very same ones that yesterday seemed "fine". Please don't let that bum you out. That's actually true for healthy people too. Sometimes people are having a jolly day at the beach, eating pizza and drinking beer (I know, who are these lucky people?!), yet suddenly they may need to run to the bathroom (we can relate, right?). They didn't suddenly get IBS, and they may well be able to turn around the next day and have pizza and beer with no issue. It happens. *For all of us, whether healing from IBS or having sudden-onset-beeline to the restroom, listen to your body. Your body is telling you something.* Your body is saying, "Hey. Not doing well right now, we need to make some changes." Interpreting what is needed is tricky, but not impossible, and listening is the key, so that we pay attention.

By the way, the pizza-and-beer on the beach gone wrong may have to do more with eating heavy carbohydrates during the heat of the day than anything else. There is a lot at play here, and I'm going to help you sort it out.

The Gastrocolic Reflex

Our bodies are a symphony of moving parts, working (or at least trying to work) in harmony with each other, to manage the wellness of our cells, our organs, our hormones and all that goes into a healthy body in an efficient and effective way. There is a lovely physiological reflex that occurs within moments of putting food into our mouths, called the gastrocolic reflex, but believe me that when I first learned of the reflex, I didn't think it was lovely at all. I thought it was the bane of my existence, the thing that was causing me to have to leave the table within a few bites of food, because here we go again, the intestines were shouting "NOW!" and I could only abide by their wishes. The reason I now think of this amazing reflex as a beautiful thing, is because I now understand how to make it work for me, not against me. We are now partners, me and GR. Here's how to understand the reflex so that you too can become allies with this mechanism, and begin to gain control of your world again.

The moment food passes the lips - possibly even before that, as when the scent of something triggers the salivary glands - the gastrocolic reflex sends a message to the intestines to initiate motility, or what is called "peristalsis". Said another way, it gets the ol' gastrointestinal tract going. Peristalsis is involuntary, meaning we don't say "Intestine, start undulating!" like we can to our fingers ("Fingers, wave hello!"). It is not something we consciously control. The gastrocolic reflex does this in order to allow you to consume more food, by way of moving the previously eaten food through the very long, very windy, very lengthy intestinal tract, and allow you to consume the calories you need to survive. Though it may not seem so, we often have up to a couple days worth of meals in transit, making their way through our body, as the amazing body absorbs what it needs to keep us healthy, full of nutrition, and feeling good. The gastrocolic reflex alone involves the autonomic nervous system, the enteric nervous system, and the cells of the gastrointestinal tract that regulate endocrine functions[8]. It really is amazing.

---

[8]

https://www.ncbi.nlm.nih.gov/books/NBK549888/#:~:text=The%20gastr ocolic%20reflex%20is%20a,with%20the%20ingestion%20of%20food.

People with IBS have been shown to have a stronger gastrocolic reflex[9], meaning the response to the food trigger is faster, which can cause the urgent need to use the bathroom even though we've literally taken only a few bites. This stronger response can be the cause of the pain, bloating, and gas that is often associated with IBS, because things are moving very fast, possibly before they are "ready" to move to the next stage of the railroad track I think of as my intestinal journey. This is true whether you tend toward IBS-D or IBS-C. The gastrocolic reflex can still attempt to move things along, even when constipated, which can cause a "charley horse" type feeling in the colon, when the muscles spasm painfully. Likewise, with IBS-D, there may be a similar sensation of a spasm when the colon is clamping down repeatedly.

Some foods have been shown to trigger the gastrocolic reflex much more than others. These foods are considered to have a strong gastrocolic reflex, or to be higher on the GR index, whereas other foods, less likely to trigger a strong response, would be considered a low GR index. Make note, even the foods that are lower still trigger the reflex; they just do so in a way that is calmer, and therefore, much more pleasant for we humans experiencing it.

If you're thinking you can just quit reading here, and start eating only foods with a low GR, remember that our digestion is a veritable symphony of processes, and there's a bit more to it than just plucking out one melody. It might sound nice for a while, but the chances of your body being able to operate as a fully functioning orchestra by playing only one small part won't last. Let's take a little more time with the concept of the GR, with some examples of how different foods might impact it.

---

[9]

https://www.ncbi.nlm.nih.gov/books/NBK549888/#:~:text=The%20gastrocolic%20reflex%20has%20correlations,diarrhea%2C%20bloating%2C%20and%20tenesmus.

Understanding Food Choices

There are so many factors that go into the health-giving properties of foods. When we think of a fruit, let's say an apple, the nutrient breakdown is calculated in each individual category - this much fiber, these many vitamins, this much sugar. But the reality is that **our bodies make use of the available nutrients in different ways, depending on *how* we consume the foods, in its whole state or in a highly processed state.** When we eat an apple, just the act of breaking the peel, taking a crunchy first bite into the meaty pulp, and beginning that chewing process activates a ton of mechanisms in our bodies, like getting our salivary glands going, which send messages to the rest of our digestive system to get ready, and triggering the gastrocolic reflex that food is coming. The act of chewing also breaks down the food, allowing our body to begin the recognition of the various nutrients for absorption. That peel that always gets stuck in our teeth? Even that keeps our dental health optimized, via the natural "floss" and getting up under those gums in ways that soft, over-processed foods just don't do for us. The fiber in the apple not only gives the body a wonderful digestive tool for keeping our vital intestines healthy and functioning, but also helps the body offset the sugars in the apple, that without the fiber, are processed differently than with. The eating of a whole apple (not meaning the entire thing, but meaning eating it in its whole, natural state) has a very different effect on the body than, say, drinking a glass of apple juice, or even eating applesauce. This is important to understand for health overall, but also for IBS specifically, because we can't say that an apple, for example, has a "low GR index" or a "high GR index", because it depends entirely on how we consume it. Make sense? Understanding just a few more pieces can help bring this all together in a way that is manageable. Stick with me.

Transit Time

Transit time is hugely important with IBS and widely misunderstood. **Everybody processes food a little bit differently with different foods, and importantly, you may experience things differently some days than you do other days, for the same food.** This is not intended to be discouraging, but rather to help free you from thinking each and every meal will have an immediate impact that you will be able to say "Yes, that is a safe food always", or "No, that food will never work again". Most of the time, unless you have an allergy to a food, it's not going to work like that, and you can be glad it's not! Now that I have found my way out of the pendulum swingin' reactive response to my inflamed intestines and anxiety, I can eat pretty much anything within reason, because I now understand the big picture. Side note - I don't eat greasy cheeseburgers and chocolate shakes just because I can, though. I still choose health-first; I have way more variety than I did when healing from IBS, and a lot less forethought is needed when I choose my meals.

Transit time is the time it takes food to make its way through the body, from mouth to out. Some things you can eat and your body might be able to break them down, and move them through your system towards elimination much more quickly than other kinds of foods. Because of this, it's entirely possible that you may not experience symptoms of certain foods until possibly even a couple days later. Some foods, you may have symptoms within an hour, or even within minutes. I know when I was in my own personal hell, it was usually the moment I swallowed - that old digestive engine revved up and kept revving. This makes it remarkably difficult - dare I say impossible - to truly identify your reactions to foods. It made it seem like every. single. thing. I ate was causing me to have an issue, and in a way, it was. But, it wasn't that the foods were the issue - it was that I hadn't yet gotten my system to calm down enough to trust that some foods just didn't need the engine revved to that degree. My body was on high

31

alert, my intestines likely very irritated, inflamed, and unable to distinguish the correct response needed to process variety.

Transit time can be impacted by food combinations. What I mean is that let's say you are having a hard time with cheese (moves through you like lightning with lots of thunder), and you have no issue at all with potatoes (just a leisurely walk in the park), but you eat a baked potato with cheese. Can you see how you might not be able to identify "the problem"? And, what if you also ate that loaded spud after or during a particularly stressful day? Or your day became stressful as you ate. The very good news is that *you don't have to identify each individual food that "works" or doesn't.* There is another, better, safer way, which I promise I will be sharing with you very soon.

Allergy vs Intolerance

We often use, in both the IBS and greater dietary world, these terms interchangeably. They are not. **An *allergy* is something that has pretty distinctive adverse effects, and should be taken seriously, whereas an *intolerance* is more of a nuisance, but could possibly develop into an allergy if you continue to assault your body with things it doesn't like.** Think of it this way: if you get stung by a bee, *and you are not allergic, you will be uncomfortable for a while*, whereas *if you are allergic to the bee, you may swell up like a balloon and may even need to be rushed to the ER.* If you are not allergic to a bee sting, but get stung by a bee over and over and over and over, you could likely end up with more severe issues, and could possibly even develop an immune response (an allergy) over time, to bee stings. Now, I love bees, really and truly, but my point here is that if every teacher who took students on a field trip were told that all the students were **allergic** to bees, because they hurt when they got stung, that would really be misinformation for the teacher and possibly cause a lot of panic and undue stress when they visited the botanical gardens in May.

So speaking accurately is important, in life, in general, and certainly when speaking about your health, and your IBS symptoms. If you are saying you are allergic to something, but you are not truly allergic, shift to "intolerant". This may let you shift to "moderately intolerant", to "I just have to be careful with that", to "it used to bother me a lot when my IBS was out of control, but now I can eat it just fine."

An intolerance is something your body just doesn't tolerate well. Maybe you just don't feel so good from it. An allergy is something that your body actually has a response to, like an inflammatory response which means your immune system is revving up to combat an invader. Gluten is one of those things where people are finding that they're allergic to gluten, which is generally associated with celiac disease. Many people with IBS (diagnosed, or un-diagnosed and wondering) are questioning whether they have a gluten issue. An intolerance to gluten means maybe your body just doesn't break it down or process it very well, (and remember you might not see that response until a couple of days later), so it's very hard to know if it is truly gluten that you are intolerant to. For a gluten allergy, there are specific tests that can be done. If you don't have the allergy, and are just suspecting (wondering, hoping to determine) whether gluten is the culprit causing your woes, stay with me. There is quite possibly a clearer path for you.

Common Culprits

There are certain foods that could be culprits for digestive issues that you may wish to consider avoiding for a period of time, and then introducing back into your diet slowly and carefully to be sure you're not dealing with an allergy. **They are: corn, wheat,**

33

gluten, eggs, dairy, yeast, peanuts, soy, and sugar.[10] For IBS, you will want to also consider removing processed foods (pretty much anything with an ingredients list) from your diet, until you have a good strong handle on what you can tolerate, or, until you can tolerate foods again, once your body heals. **It's entirely possible that as time goes on, and you get better and healthier and stronger, that there will be fewer and fewer foods that you find to be possible irritants or that cause any digestive issue.** *That is one of the most wonderful aspects of this journey back to wellness that I did not suspect, and in fact, would never have believed possible.* My hope is that you are able to discover the same thing.

---

[10]

https://books.google.com/books/about/GI_Janel_Permanent_IBS_SIBO_Resolution.html?id=6q_YyQEACAAJ

The Syndrome of the Irritable Bowel

What the heck is it? **Irritable Bowel Syndrome is exactly that - a syndrome, which is a category of illness or un-wellness that describes a group of symptoms occurring together.** In some cases, it might be an irritable bowel, which can have no discernible laboratory tests to definitely say "this is IBS". Other syndromes may have a test, like for Downs syndrome. The "syndrome" part indicates there are a group of signs and symptoms characterizing the condition.

IBS is a *disorder*, not a disease. This is important to note, because of the way it is diagnosed, which is by <u>ruling out</u> other possibilities. Because there are other disorders in the world that can overlap or coincide with IBS, making a definitive diagnosis can be complicated.

IBS is considered a *functional* disorder, referring to how the brain and the body communicate. *It does not mean you are doing something wrong. It does not mean that it's all in your head (it's not).* Other functional disorders include fibromyalgia, chronic pelvic pain, and more. Each of these recognize that the body's processes are impaired, but medical or scientific detection of what is causing the condition is typically not possible.

"A **functional disorder** is a medical condition that impairs normal functioning of bodily processes that remains largely undetected under examination, dissection or even under a microscope. At the exterior, there is no appearance of abnormality. This stands in contrast to a **structural disorder** (in which some part of the body can be seen to be abnormal) or a psychosomatic disorder (in which symptoms are caused by psychological or psychiatric illness). Definitions vary somewhat between fields of medicine.

Generally, the mechanism that causes a functional disorder is unknown, poorly understood, or occasionally unimportant for treatment purposes. The brain or nerves are often believed to be involved. It is common that a person with one functional disorder will have others."[11]

The Bountiful Array of IBS Symptoms

The gut and the brain don't interact correctly or as expected with IBS. This can result in sensitivity in the gut (in the actual intestines), and also affect how the muscles that control digestion contract (peristalsis). There may be pain in the abdomen, bloating, and either chronic or extreme diarrhea (IBS-D) or constipation (IBS-C) or both (IBS-M).

For those who experience IBS-D, there can be urgency (like most diarrhea events, right!) and frequency. It can happen every fifteen minutes, and go on for a few hours. If you have diarrhea once a month, that's probably not IBS, but if it's pretty common - I believe the medical model is ¼ of your bathroom experiences are diarrhea

---

[11] https://en.wikipedia.org/wiki/Functional_disorder

(or constipation, or both), then you would fit one of the criteria for identifying whether you have IBS.

Beyond the well-known and unpleasant bowel movement issues, over the many years that I experienced unexplained digestive issues, I experienced a wide variety of other symptoms. Not everyone has the same symptoms, but I list these in case you wonder if you're imagining things, or if you have a bunch of different things going on. At times I was sure I had terminal illnesses on top of a messed up gut. In my experience and in my opinion, when our gut is out of whack, there is a wide-ranging array of symptoms that can result, Including:

Audible noises from my abdomen. This was so embarrassing. *Remember the scenes from the Titanic when the ship was sinking, and the moans of the ship as it sunk? That's what it sounded like for me.* Or like Dory imitating the whale, from Finding Nemo. It can also be gurgles, and what sounds like passing gas, though it's bubbles popping inside the abdomen (not exiting). These audible sounds seemed to be the first sign that things were awry for me. Rather than being unduly embarrassed, I now take it as a sign that something is getting out of whack, and I need to make a change.

Feeling nauseated. This can happen around food. It can happen around using the bathroom. I sometimes woke up in the morning feeling that way. I have woken up at night feeling like I'm going to vomit. I know people who do. Nearly always when I was able to pass gas or stool, the nausea went away.

Bloating can be a big symptom (ha ha). I would eat something, or even drink something, and my tummy would swell up like a balloon, so full and hard, almost immediately. It could have been a party trick, it was so reliable. "Watch this!"

I experienced at times extreme weight loss, which is understandable, given that during many periods of the experience food was going right through me, and oddly, I also experienced periods of weight gain. I believe that was related to trying different food combinations, and I wondered too if my body was trying to retain fuel, like a bear getting ready for winter, thanks to my bouts of not being able to get much nutrition from the food flying through me.

Feelings of lethargy and fatigue were also common. I was just exhausted, from the physical and mental and emotional strain of the disorder, but also, I believe, from my body trying so hard to heal. We need rest to heal. Our bodies work hard for us, and downtime is critical to allow optimal healing. I certainly didn't take that time for years.

I've mentioned the anxiety, the added stress, and, certainly I experienced depression. I would wonder if the stress caused the IBS or if the IBS was caused by the anxiety, but it didn't really matter. Depression is a pretty understandable evolution of this cycle, and can be dangerous. Please, take it seriously. Address it.[12]

Other weird symptoms I had that I really wondered whether they were related include:

Foot pain, leg pain: It was so consistent at times, and would occur during the time in the bathroom. I believe it was related to nerve issues, since the nerves were all jangled up and sending out rather desperate impulses. That has resolved completely for me, and I now believe it was related to the psoas muscle (discussed later in this book).

Belly button bulge: This was terrifying. There were a few times I felt the oddest bulge near my belly button, and could actually see it pulsing - it was my heart beating, and I could see something pressing out of my abdomen. I believe it was the intestinal sphincter that meets the stomach, and with so much bloating and

---

[12] https://www.cdc.gov/reproductivehealth/depression/resources.htm

pressure, it was, literally, bulging. I did find ways to soothe it after the first couple of times it happened. A warm rice heating pad was wonderful, and actually laying my hands on the bulge and calming myself also helped. I have read of others who have described similar symptoms.

Bleeding: TMI, I know. This was also terrifying. If you experience bleeding, be sure to consult with your trusted health practitioner. Oddly, mine were never very concerned about it - they felt it was "hemorrhoids" which was strange to me, because I wasn't ever (like, EVER) constipated.

Poor quality nails and hair: Particularly during times of weight loss, I noticed my nails were very brittle, and I would lose more hair in the shower or on my brush. This makes perfect sense to me - I wasn't retaining really any nutritional content as food was just galloping through me, so of course my hair and nails were impacted by the lack of vitamin and mineral intake. It's another good thing to pay attention to know when you must make changes.

Low-grade fever: I would also sometimes have a fever. I don't believe it was related to infection, as it was low-grade, and the numerous stool tests I did never came back with any bacteria or parasites. It would always resolve on its own after a short time and may have had nothing to do with IBS or my digestive issues. It's possible that the extreme fatigue I had resulted in a low grade fever.

Why Are There So Many Digestive Issues in the World Today?

I've seen varying statistics over the years about the prevalence of digestive issues in the world, including 20% of Americans complaining of gastrointestinal distress, and an alarming 1 in every 3 adults in the world having a GI issue. I don't know how accurate those claims are, and statistics on the web change quickly, but a quick Google search reveals:

- For every ten adults in the world, four suffer from functional gastrointestinal disorders of varying severity. This is shown by a study of more than 73,000 people in 33 countries. University of Gothenburg scientists are among those now presenting these results.[13]
- According to a new, national survey of more than 2,000 U.S. adults, 72 percent said they have experienced at least one gastrointestinal (GI) symptom a few times a month or more.[14]
- Whether it's a meal that doesn't agree with us or a lingering gastrointestinal ailment requiring lifestyle changes and treatment, digestive problems are extremely common, afflicting as many as one in five Americans.[15]
- Irritable Bowel Syndrome is the single most common chronic health disorder in America, Canada, the UK, Australia, and New Zealand.[16]
- IBS affects more people than asthma, diabetes, and depression **combined**.[17]

Clearly, there are digestive problems in the world, but the question is, why?

13

https://www.gu.se/en/news/four-of-ten-adults-worldwide-have-functional-gastrointestinal-disorders
14

https://news.abbvie.com/news/new-survey-reveals-more-than-half-americans-are-living-with-gastrointestinal-symptoms-and-not-seeking-care-from-doctor.htm#:~:text=6%2C%202013%20%2FPRNewswire%2F%20%2D%2D,unexplained%20weight%2Dloss%20and%20non%2D

15 https://www.tanner.org/the-scope/6-common-digestive-disorders

16 https://www.betterhealthusa.com/public/318.cfm

17 https://www.ncbi.nlm.nih.gov/pmc/articles/PMC3921083/

There are a lot of different theories about what causes IBS, and why there is such a prevalence of not only irritable bowel syndrome, but other functional disorders, as well as an abundance of other digestive issues. **A common theory is that people who suffer from IBS experienced some type of trauma in their lives that "set it off" or even started it, like a surgery, or a heavy duty dose of antibiotics, or maybe a parasite or a food poisoning.** The thought is that something threw everything out of whack initially, and the illness or syndrome progressed. I don't know if it's true, but it seems plausible that an event (or events) occurred that knocked that balance out of whack, and the body, for whatever reason, just wasn't able to regain homeostasis. I have certainly had some traumas like the ones listed.

I also believe it's possible that *some people are prone to processing their emotions and their stress in their guts.* We used to say (back in the olden days) that some people had a "nervous nature", and while we don't necessarily label people like this anymore, it seems reasonable to me that it's the same idea of some people getting headaches. I do still hear people say that so-and-so has "a nervous stomach", which is used to explain why someone may have digestive issues, though of course, it doesn't really explain anything.

I firmly believe it's worth considering that **our food sources have changed dramatically in even just a couple of generations.** I think it's possible that the surge in IBS worldwide could be partially related to the genetically modified food that we're seeing in our lives. We also have an influx of certain kinds of food in our diet that we get hit with, from all sides, like soy, corn, and wheat, which are used as fillers in so many of our products. I am not condemning modified foods, but I do think that the scientific community doesn't really know for sure the long-term effects. I am not condemning soy, corn, or wheat, but I do think too much of any one thing isn't good.

I also believe the digestive issues could be due, in part, to an overexposure to toxins related to the increased levels of pesticides, herbicides, and other poisons used in massive agriculture to produce perfect foods. I am aware that these chemicals are approved for use by the scientists who study them, but I also know that we are exposed to a great deal more toxins than could ever be analyzed or proven "safe", and over a much longer term than could actually be studied. It's worth considering that there is an environmental aspect to this syndrome, not to make us feel doomed or that things are out of our control, but rather to be open to the possibilities that things may need to change.

I have a suspicion that the copious amount of plastics in our air, water, and ultimately, our bodies, may also play a role in the state of our health. A recent study found that the average American consumes one credit-card-size amount of plastic **each week**[18]. This again is not intended to portend doom or an inability to manage our health. Not at all; we are not victims unless we choose to be. This suspicion is shared because in my opinion we must recognize the possible effects of our current lifestyle, as a society, as well as our own individual choices, so that we can make changes, as individuals, as a society, sooner rather than later. It is not too late, and I firmly believe change **can** happen for the good of our planet, and our future.

Whatever the reason for IBS, or any of the functional disorders or GI issues in the world, there are steps we **can** take. As individuals caring for our own bodies, we can choose to wash our foods, try to purchase items without plastic packaging, recycle, and learn more about legislation that impacts our food sources and our planet. We, as a society, can also support organic agriculture, vote for protections of our water sources, and encourage retailers to forego plastics (plastic bags, plastic take-out containers, and plastic straws

---

18

https://www.cnn.com/2022/10/31/us/microplastic-credit-card-per-week/index.html#:~:tex t=Here's%20something%20that%20will%20haunt,A%20credit%20card!

are all great places to start!). None of this needs to feel like a burden, or weigh you down. We can approach these efforts with eagerness, and hope, and a gratefulness that we are so fortunate to be able to make choices for the wellbeing of ourselves and our fellow living beings on this beautiful earth.

I believe it's possible to heal from IBS, with patience, diligence, and kindness. **We've got to be kind to ourselves as we move through this, treating our body with love and care, and our emotions as valid, and our concerns with positive action.** I hope to help you with each of these. We don't really know the "cause" of a lot of things that people suffer through, despite what we might like to believe. We know things that cause issues, but even then, not everyone is going to get the illness that is "caused" by whatever food or behavior or genetic trait they partake in or have. Not every smoker gets cancer; not every yoga-practicing vegetarian avoids a terminal condition. **There is one thing that does have a known physical impact that you do have a great deal of potential control over, one that you may not pay enough attention to, and that is stress.**

The Incredible Cycle of Stress

The stress of IBS is very real. It manifests within the body in a multitude of ways. Whether we are having an *episode* (flare up), or are nervous that we are going to have an episode, the roles stress and anxiety play are multifaceted and should not be dismissed. This is an extremely important aspect of your wellness that is often dealt with "last", after focusing on the "more important" symptoms first (getting through a morning without agonizing pain, fear, anxiety, or embarrassment). Stress can cause the muscles to tense, and you may hold that tension in various parts of your body without even knowing it. You may hold it in your abdomen, in your shoulders, your neck, your posture, your low back. I used to, unknowingly, clench my fists and hold my breath, creating even more tension in my body. This tension alone can cause painful conditions that you may worry and wonder if they are related to or a cause of your IBS, or something else, causing even more tension and stress. The wondering and worrying is really hell. Think of the COVID pandemic - many people experienced symptoms that no one was sure if they were related to or caused by the coronavirus, or if it was "something else". "Oh my gosh, my hands are tingling! Is it related?" We can become so preoccupied with mysterious states of ill health that "everything" seems to be related. It makes it very hard to sort out where to even begin.

Please note that considering whether a strange symptom may or may not be related to a serious illness does not make a person paranoid. We are flooded with snippets of information about diseases, and our news outlets intentionally create attention-grabbing headlines to get readers and clicks. We are often told of dangers in 30-second or one or two minute sound bites. Very rarely will that allow for the big picture or all the facts to be presented. It is normal to feel a bit in the dark, to not know or feel confident about the "what if" possibilities of what may be happening to us. The very best approach to offset this media hype and incomplete information is to take the time to learn what you can, get the bigger picture, gather support around you of informed individuals who also take the time to learn the big picture, and trust your inner knowing.

When you are stressed, your emotions are impacted. **You simply feel different emotionally. You may be quick to anger, near tears, or conversely, find yourself shutting down. Stress and your emotions can also have an effect on your physical body.** They can impact your respiratory system, causing you to breathe shallowly, rapidly, or even to constrict the airways. Restricted breathing can cause panic attacks. When you are stressed (whether in the moment or over a long period of your time) your heart rate can increase, and your stress hormones are elevated, which, over periods of prolonged stress, can increase your risk for cardiovascular issues. Perhaps most importantly, there is research showing that stress can cause inflammation in the body, which can lead to chronic health conditions.[19]

I'm sure you've heard of "inflammation", which can be the body's response to fighting something in the moment, or something we may call "acute" (an itchy rash is an inflamed response that indicates the body is dealing with an invader, perhaps poison ivy). In the case of long-term or ongoing (i.e., chronic) inflammation, the body's response is to see potentially everything as a possible invader, and it runs on high to combat all the things it perceives it has to contend with. Our modern world provides us with ample,

---

19

https://www.everydayhealth.com/wellness/united-states-of-stress/link-betw een-stress-inflammation/#:~:text=Research%20shows%20that%20stress%2 0can,number%20of%20chronic%20health%20conditions.

and ongoing, opportunities to be stressed, to experience stress, and to stay in a heightened state of stress, (even without the stress of IBS!) Our phones for example are forever messing with our hormones, exciting us, angering us, calling to us, beckoning us, or when silent, stressing us out that something is terribly wrong![20] **Most of the modern world doesn't have real predators at their heels, but most of us live in our bodies as if we do.** Granted, there are real threats, but the body's innate response to danger is now firing nearly all our waking moments, in situations that are not really truly dangerous, *creating a stress cycle that, if left unchecked, is very, very hard on our bodies over time.*

All of this scary information is to emphasize the importance of getting a handle on your stress even when you don't have a syndrome that is stressful. This is not the item to skip over. You must make time for it. You must not shelve it "until" you get the other symptoms under control. It IS the symptom to get under control. You can find relief from the physically harrowing symptoms much more quickly and with less guess work if you also incorporate stress-reducing measures. Although I believe my path to wellness was relatively fast (once I got on the right track) in the big picture of the decades that I suffered, I also believe that I would have been able to identify solutions more quickly, with less guess work, and more easily, had I placed more importance and effort on lowering my stress levels first, or even in conjunction with my other efforts.

20

https://physicianoneurgentcare.com/blog/the-link-between-cell-phone-use-anxiety-depression/#:~:text=Nearly%205%20billion%20people%20use,technology%20to%20escape%20from%20stress.

What Worked and Why

Here's what you came for, but please, please please if you skipped to this and didn't read the stuff before it, understand you are missing out on some critical elements that helped me tremendously. If the information you skipped could move your healing along even more quickly, isn't it worth a read?

The funny thing about my journey back to health is that I already knew a lot of this stuff, right, because I'm a holistic wellness coach, and I have spent a lot of years helping others find balance in their lives. *But knowing something and actually applying it, embracing it, is a very different experience than teaching or coaching about it.* It was only once I shifted my focus from magnifying each and every morsel I ate and the immediate after-effect (which is a no-win and will lead you down multiple rabbit holes), to the bigger, broader picture of my overall health and my desire to feel *better* that things began to really shift for me. I just wanted to feel better. That was the end game, and keeping my eye on that prize was critical to this happily ever after I have now.

The Freedom Framework, Revisited

As you take in the information I am about to share in this section, please recall the three basic principles of the Freedom Framework. Remember that it is much easier to allow, versus push against, to be forgiving of our choices instead of speaking harshly in our minds, to be kinder, just a little bit kinder, as we navigate the many paths each day brings us. Trying a slightly kinder thought, a little less resistant path, a little more allowing decision, will open you to the easier and better and kinder and happier choice each moment can offer you. You may be thinking this doesn't have a thing to do with

47

your current digestive issues, that you do not "choose" to feel so unwell. The choice, my friend, is in how you perceive your experience, how you imagine your journey to wellness, how you relate to your body, how you talk about your desires to be healed.

The three main points of the Freedom Framework again are:

1. Striving for the next better thing [emotion, food, thought, experience, relationship, job, choice, decision]. Always.

2. Embracing what is unique to YOU, and understanding WHY. What is right for the masses is not necessarily right for the individual.

3. Mastering continued growth! Understanding what is right for you in the moment will inevitably change as you continue to evolve, and as life continues to shift!

The Freedom Framework not only applies to your relationship with your decisions around food and your physical health, it applies to and works with relationships to others, with self-care, with every choice you have to make and with every thought you think, to bring you to a better, happier, easier, healthier existence. It works because you will grow to understand:

- Intuitively what the next best choice is for you
- Why it is the best choice in the moment for you
- That there is no failure, no going backward, no keeping score, no guilt, and no shame
- What is best for you specifically; not for "everyone" or "most people", but for YOU
- That life happens (conflict, hardship, curveballs, travel, sickness, happy events, hard events, boring events), and

you will be ready and armed with the knowledge of how to proceed with health, ease, and happiness

Keep these tenets in mind as you learn new information, and open yourself to trying new ways of looking at your options to wellness.

My Turning Point:
The Ultimate Gut Reset

For my journey, it was a good 20-30 years of coping with IBS symptoms, depending on when we agree it started for me, in a state of up and down, of worry and preoccupation with my diet, trying different diets, like eliminating dairy, then eliminating gluten, and so on, before I was able to turn myself around for good.. I was always searching, searching for something to help me feel better. At the end there, those last horrible three years where I was in what I would call a flared state almost continually, I was just not doing well at all. I was continuing to seek medical care, seeking answers from Western medicine and alternative medicine, but no one seemed to be able to understand how bad it was, or give me any truly helpful advice. My diet had become very, very restricted. I was depressed. I had experienced a pretty extreme weight loss at certain times during those three years, and along came the food supplement I thought would save me, that actually did real damage (again, remember because I had misused it, by using way too much at once). Something had to change.

Literally every single time I ate something, within minutes - even before I could finish a meal - my body said "NOW" and off I would gallop to the bathroom. Food intake, no matter what it was, if it involved chewing, had me in a vicious, and I mean vicious cycle of my body needing to purge, immediately, and then often every fifteen minutes, urgently, for four or five bouts. And sometimes far more. Clearly I hadn't even eaten that much food if I was only bites in, but my body was on such high alert to

"ELIMINATE! ELIMINATE! ELIMINATE" that it would over-respond. I am certain there will be "experts" who disagree with this and will say that it had to be something I was eating, and I will graciously allow them this truth: It was something I was eating. It was food.

When it was that terribly bad, which it was for months and months at the end, before I finally took the reins, I was such a prisoner of my body, hungry all the time, and terrified of eating. It's incredibly freeing to me to be able to laugh about it now, but I honestly still laugh about it the same way as you do about that close call with a car accident, as you take a shaky breath and say, "Gosh, that was really something wasn't it." So, the continual small meals throughout the day, despite being the generally accepted "good" advice for IBS management, was not working for me in the least. I knew that the best I felt (which was not great, let me tell you), was when I had finally gotten through a cycle of dashing to the restroom, but was not yet heading for the next meal, and had a moment of calm. It was then that I decided to fast, and just give my poor body a break from digesting anything, that turned out to be the single best decision to start to turn things around.

Fasting in the world of IBS is generally seen as a "bad" idea, and I understand why. The theory (and it's a widely accepted theory) is that many small meals throughout the day help keep symptoms under control. For me, large meals were definitely a problem, so I agree, smaller meals, smaller portions, is a great plan. However, the ongoing food-in/run-to-the-bathroom scenario wasn't working for me. I knew that fasting was frowned upon, and at the very least, not recommended for sufferers of IBS, but at that point, I felt I had nothing to lose.

Perhaps we can look at this way. If the things we are adding are causing issues, and we can't figure out what "it" is, and "it" seems like "everything", doesn't it make sense to just stop? For a little while? And let the poor intestinal tract take a much-needed break?

I now think of it as a Gut Reset. I wish I would have done this so much sooner. I wish I wouldn't have waited until I was in such a terrible state.

Understand that this is not fasting for weight loss. This is not intermittent fasting. This is not for ketosis, or blood sugar, or anything other than being very kind to a possibly very worn out and inflamed digestive system.

For me, I felt better immediately. I fasted for four days the first time. I don't think that long is necessarily needed for everyone, but I needed it, and I felt fantastic for every day of it, because it was such a welcome relief of the hell I had been living through. How you feel during a fast is a good indicator of how well it's working, for this purpose. What I mean by "fasting" is I took in only liquids, and only clean liquids, which were (and continue to be, whenever I fast) bone broth, which is very, very soothing, very comforting, and very nourishing; water, plain, or sometimes with a little bit of lemon juice; and herbal teas. I have also sometimes added rice water, which is super soothing for me (again, this is not for ketosis, or your blood sugar, or weight loss - it is about soothing the organs). I knew I tolerated rice well, so I felt I would do just fine with rice water, and it added just a touch of sustenance that helped get me through some of the moments of gnawing hunger (which always pass within about 20 minutes anyway). The bone broth and rice water were warm and soothing and felt that they added some sustenance, the lemon water was cool (not cold) and refreshing, and the warm (not hot) teas were comforting and soothing. We'll talk about temperatures a little later, but that's important to note - extremes in temperature can throw you off course as well.

Although that first fast was a long four days, and when I say four days, I do mean 96 hours, I felt only better, and better, and better. I felt tired, I felt a little headachy sometimes, but I also felt moments of physical energy, and certainly clarity in my mind, and most of all, **my poor belly** was finally at peace.

Emotionally, I felt such joy at the reprieve from my fixation and preoccupation with my gut, I probably would have kept going, if not for an unexpected jolt back into consuming "food" that was not at all planned (and why I use the term "food" loosely you will soon understand). I would have really liked to ease back into eating healthy food a different way than I did, but as it happened, at the end of the four days I was heading into an MRI of my abdomen that little did I know I would have to drink some kind of metal liquid dye. Ugh! My poor body. What a radical shift from the calm and peace of fasting with such wonderful liquids, to the jarring introduction of a metal dye!

And once again, the moment I consumed it, I was back on the carousel, only, this time, I had a little bit more time in between the bouts. The metal dye did trigger my gastrocolic reflex, but not as extremely as I had been living with for those many long months prior.. I only had to ask the technicians to let me out of the MRI machine once, (though the entire time I was in the big machine I was terrified I would have to get out of there quickly). I was immediately back into that fear - that awful anxiety, but still…the whole experience was so revealing, that even after consuming such an awful "food" after days of being so kind to my gut, I didn't go into a complete and total nose-dive. I did, after the MRI, feel I wanted to put something kinder than metal into my belly, and so I broke that fast officially and started again with foods, without a very clear path of what to introduce first or how, but even with my bumpy reintroduction into the world of eating, I knew I was onto something.

A week later, I fasted again, this time for 2 and a half days. I had the same immediate calm, and such emotional relief, and, this time, I planned what I would introduce as my first foods after coming out of it. Over my next few forays of short fasts and then reintroducing food, I made some mistakes with what to introduce and when, how soon, in what order, but after four separate fasting episodes over a couple of months for the purpose of a Gut Reset, I got it down to a true and total reset. That's when things really turned the corner for me - I started to really be able to choose differently, to really figure out what and how to eat while my body healed.

Now, you might think four days of fasting should be ample time to heal, or 4 separate resets should have been enough, but let me ask you: *if you had been continually punched in the arm, every single time you ate, for years, and then eventually, four days goes by without being punched, do you think that when you first eat again, and the arm is punched, it will be completely healed?* Or do you think it could still be sore? **Healing takes time.** *Those intestines are amazing and hearty, but those tissues take time to heal.* **You are, after all, only human.**

Even as I continued to improve, if I had any setbacks, or just felt I was teetering on the verge of not doing so well, I would fast again, perhaps about once a month, for the first year of my journey back to wellness. I now do what ends up being roughly a 36 hour fast, and might look like dinner on a Sunday night, then I won't eat anything at all on Monday, and I won't eat again until I break my fast Tuesday morning. It has continued to help a lot, over the course of the months of my recovery, and I now look forward to it, even though I don't really "have" to do it out of necessity anymore. It feels like a nice gift I am giving to my wonderful digestive system, my wonderful organs that work so hard for me, my ever vigilant soldiers.

Now a word of warning. There's a lot of fasting information out there. There's intermittent fasting, 5-and-2 fasting, and on it goes. I want to emphasize again that I'm not talking about fasting for the purpose of weight loss. I'm not talking about fasting for blood sugar, or to put you into ketosis, or any other purpose than to **give your digestive system a break**. I mention this because as you look up information about fasting, many of them may say that it's fine to have coffee during your fast, and it's even fine to put cream in it, but anything that your body really needs to actively digest, I steer clear of. The closest I come to putting in something to "digest" is the rice water. Remember too that coffee has caffeine, and it's also rather greasy, both of which can be gastro stimulants. This is just one example of something that might be allowed on "other" fasts for other purposes, that you may want to steer clear of for the purposes of a Gut Reset.

It's important that if you have concerns about fasting, if you are underweight or anemic or have other health issues, or if you have any concerns that a fast could make things worse, consult with your trusted practitioner. It's also very important to understand with fasting that you shouldn't feel sicker. If you feel sicker during a fast, break the fast with something kind and gentle to ease you back into food. Check out Appendix A for what I drink when I do my Gut Reset fasting.

Learning How to Eat

Whether or not you decide to fast and do a Gut Reset to let your digestive system settle down or not, there are some truths I've learned about eating with IBS. The following information will help inform you of how to eat going forward in your life, and also, what foods you might consider breaking your fast with, in the event you do decide to do a Gut Reset. The information to follow works for both.

Soluble vs Insoluble Fiber

Whether you are adding food after a fast, as part of an elimination diet, or even just making a shift in your eating habits to aid your body in healing from IBS, there is one known truth that the greater IBS community (medical and non-medical) seems to support: *soluble fiber is key*. I'm going to break this down for you in an easy to understand and easy to follow way, so that you can start feeling better right away.

There are different kinds of fiber in fruits and vegetables: soluble fiber and insoluble fiber. A lot of foods have both insoluble and soluble. "Soluble" means this kind of fiber can be broken down by water. "Insoluble" means that it takes more than just water, or is a little more difficult or challenging to break down. Put another way, **insoluble fiber is less easily digested than soluble fiber.** With soluble fiber foods, your body doesn't have to work quite so hard. They digest, or they break down a little more easily. That doesn't make insoluble fibers bad - on the contrary, they add needed bulk, and are equally important to our diets.

When you are at the doctor's office or read an article in a health magazine, were instructed to "add fiber", what is often missing from that information for those of us with IBS is that it's got to be a mix of both kinds of fiber, but here's the key: we must eat the soluble fiber *first*. **While you are healing, the very best approach seems to be to always, always, always eat soluble fiber first. Make sure that hits your belly before anything else.** Why? Remember that gastrocolic reflex we talked about earlier? When the soluble fiber is first to enter the digestive system, the body tends to respond more calmly, revving up its response in a more reasonable manner, because it doesn't see anything particularly difficult to deal with. When insoluble fiber hits the gut first, the digestive system expects to keep seeing this more complex food to be broken down, and it hits the ground running, even though that's not necessarily appropriate for the whole meal. But once that reaction starts, it takes time to get it calm again, particularly for those of us with sensitive guts.

As a general rule, to help get your mind around the kinds fibers in foods, these are a good place to start:

Root vegetables are called thusly because we eat the "root", or the part that grows in the ground - like a potato, carrot, or beet. They tend to be made up of primarily soluble fiber. The peels or rinds may be insoluble, so bear that in mind.

Our non-root veggies that are leafy, have veins, and the part we eat grows above the ground tend to be higher in insoluble fiber.

A balance between soluble fiber (typically root veggies) and insoluble fibers (typically leafy, vein-y, above the ground veggies) is key for most people. For anyone with IBS, it is widely accepted that eating some soluble fiber first is the route to a calm gut, though integrating insoluble fiber is also important. It is not a goal to eat **only** soluble fiber. *The goal is to reach a balance of both kinds of fiber, as we need them for full and balanced health.*

It took me a long time to understand that my go-to vegetable, kale, (leafy green, with veins, grows above the ground - very high in insoluble fiber) was causing a lot of my issues. We do need an array of veggies, we do need to eat the rainbow, but I decided to pick my battles and stick with healing thyself first, and then adding more balanced nutrition. Too much soluble (potatoes, carrots, turnips) can slow the intestinal tract, whereas too much insoluble fiber (kale, spinach, lettuce) can kick it into gear (and you, along with it, as you run to the bathroom). When you have IBS-C, kicking into high gear but having a roadblock results in the pain and spasms. But once you are "clear", insoluble fiber is key to keeping things moving and in balance. Check out Appendix B for a guide on learning to recognize soluble and insoluble fiber options.

How I added soluble fiber into my meals was as I said, starting with the soluble fiber first in terms of my bites. I would have a banana at breakfast, for example, and here's another thing I found: I did not have to eat the whole banana. Just a few bites of banana or any soluble fiber helped to "set the tone" for the gut response, to say, "here comes friendly food! All is well" and go from there. After my banana, or my half of a banana, I could safely have something else (within reason). Lunch might look like a few bites of cooked beets as my first bites, and then on to a salad (if I was doing very well, because that's a lot of insoluble fiber), or perhaps a rice-based salad if I needed to be a little more gentle (white rice is soluble fiber) Even if you don't plan to fast or do any kind of elimination diet, you could consider starting with adding the soluble fiber right out of the gate. **Just adding soluble fiber as the first thing when eating, and testing whether that alone makes a difference and helps calm the gut may bring some freedom!** Check out Appendix D for how I incorporated fiber depending on how I was feeling.

Fats

During one week of my particularly bad years, before I had my breakthrough with the Gut Reset, I was at a huge conference, staying in a hotel in Boston. I had already anticipated that there was no way I'd be able to join the others in the dining areas for breakfast, as the mornings were the hardest for me. I had planned to bring some soluble fiber, like instant rice I could cook in the microwave, and when I arrived on the Sunday afternoon prior to the conference's actual start, I walked the many blocks to a Trader Joe's and bought some rice, as well as cans of raw, preservative-free coconut milk, thinking it would be the calmest non-dairy thing with some nutrition and needed calories I could tolerate.

I found out very quickly that something wasn't right with my plan. The mornings were worse than ever, to the point that I wondered if I had a virus or flu. My days consisted of trying not to be late to the morning sessions, close to panicking at the thought of sitting in a large room with others, a bathroom nowhere in sight, self-consciously excusing myself from lunch to go drink broth back in my room and frantically scouring the internet for some truth, something that could help me figure out what I was doing wrong. I managed to attend the afternoon sessions, but was so hyper-tuned into my belly that I missed a lot of what was even being taught, afraid I would have to dash out and interrupt the trainer, and possibly embarrass myself. Finally at the end of each day, I could be in the safety of my room again, attempt to eat something - more rice! more broth! perhaps a banana! - and hope for a better day the next day. It was at the end of the conference, late the last night after another harrowing day before planning to fly out and having a whole new set of fears about being trapped in an airplane seat, unable to get to the restroom in a hurry, that I found something on the internet that started to make sense.

I'm a big proponent of fat, and believe we need healthy fats, like olive and avocado, but what I discovered is, if you're starting out your meal with the coconut milk, which has a really high fat content, the fat (even healthy fat) can be a gastrocolic trigger. Even though I was having my rice or my banana, I was chugging the coconut milk, and it's so high in fat, it not only wasn't being balanced out by the little bit of soluble fiber in my couple of bites of banana, but I was drinking it **very cold** and **first thing in the morning**. It was like a triple whammy of too cold, too much fat, and just plain too much to hit my gut on an empty stomach.

Other fats to consider are greasy foods, like fried potatoes or french fries. Yes, potatoes are soluble fiber, but be conscious of how they are prepared - lots of butter and sour cream could also be an issue, for the reasons of either dairy or fat!

The good news of course is I can now have coconut milk, even refreshingly cold. I still don't drink a lot of it first thing in the morning though but I will add it to my oatmeal or have it with some fruit, which is pretty luxurious after all the restrictions I had been living with, and I can definitely live with that. Appendix C has information about both fats and beverages.

Wily Things to Watch For

These are the things that were not necessarily on my radar, at all, when I was analyzing every bite and subsequent symptom. These are the deceptively impacting items to make note of, as you travel your journey to wellness.

Beverages

Nobody wants to have to give up their comforting morning chai, and certainly nobody wants to give up their coffee with the cream or the sugar. Here are a few things to consider that may help you decide if you would do well to step away from these choices while you heal.

Caffeine is a gastrocolic trigger. The cream? High in fat, possibly dairy (lactose), which when mixed with the acidity of coffee can even sometimes cause the cream to curdle. The sugar? Sugar, one of the Common Culprits we talked about earlier, creates a hormonal signal to the gut, which triggers that nerve connection in the intestines to digest.

Chai may possibly be a better choice, but watch the sugar and milk again. Plain black tea is an even better option, though it still has caffeine.

Other beverages I chose to put on pause included carbonated waters with natural flavors, as the carbonation seemed to blow me up like a balloon contrary to the insistence of my medical providers that it couldn't be related. I also eliminated anything with sweeteners (artificial or real). Even artificial sweeteners could be a culprit, because our bodies don't necessarily know that it's not real.[21]

If you find yourself having a glass or three of wine at night to calm down from a harrowing day with IBS (and I assure you, you are not alone if so), consider that while you may feel calmer in the moment, alcohol is a gut irritant even for those who don't suffer from IBS, so that's a no brainer, and I can tell you, can be pretty tough when you just want to numb the hell of IBS and dull the

---

[21] https://kids.frontiersin.org/articles/10.3389/frym.2019.00051

edges of the long, anxiety-ridden days. You'll be calmer in the long run without the added damage to your body, I assure you.

The bottom line with these comfort drinks, the ones we want to give up last (or never), is that continuing to consume these known likely offenders makes it really hard to identify what's really going on.

What if, for the sake of a possibility, the coffee is the only culprit? The one and only thing causing you discomfort? *Would you give it up then?* **When you have something every single day without fail, you may tend to say, "it can't be the chai, I have it every day, and I don't have the same symptoms every day".** *There's flawed logic in that, because your body is constantly striving for balance and you are putting a wide variety of other things into the equation that could be having a significant effect.*

You can do this, if you decide to eliminate these comfort beverages as a possibility. You can get rid of the coffee, you can treat your body with care, you can awake and have a lovely cup of herbal gentleness, at least while you are healing. **I know a lot of these changes can be really tough, but remember your long game - if you had to eliminate coffee for three months, or even six months, and feel better** *for the rest of your life* **(meaning you get to start drinking coffee again after you feel better), wouldn't that be worth it?**

Appendix C has information about both fats and beverages.

Timing/Time of Day
As I climbed over the hump from feeling terrible most of the time to feeling okay more often, intermixed with moments of not so great, I would sometimes be so frustrated that I had "fallen back" again, into a bad morning or a bad day, without really knowing

what I had done differently. Remember that what your body may respond to in the morning or when you first get up may be a totally different response than later in the day. It might not be the food choice, or the temperature; it might be that you can't have it first thing in the morning.

For example, I found after some weeks of my Gut Resets, that I could have a coconut milk smoothie in the afternoon with banana and some blueberries, and feel so good and full and satisfied, and not have an issue. I was so excited to try it as a change to what were becoming very boring breakfast choices, but when I tried that very same thing in the morning , I was right back into a hyper-responsive digestive event. Why? The extreme temperature and fat *first in the morning*. My body had healed enough to tolerate the fat from the coconut milk and the cold later in the day, after I had taken other things into my body, but to start my day with those items was too much of a shock to hit my gut with first thing.

Temperature

Remember the cold coconut milk I was guzzling at my conference? It wasn't just the fat - it was that I had it in the minifridge and it was blissfully ice cold. But the bliss was short lived when the cold alone sent my digestive engine to revving on overdrive, let alone the addition of the fats. Cold temperatures particularly, but even hot, can cause issues. In fact, now that my body digests and requests to eliminate in a very normal, well-balanced way, on the rare occasion I must get out of the house earlier than usual, and my intestines may need a little encouragement to get things moving off their normal schedule, I have found a few swallows of ice cold water works nicely to kick things into motion.

Moderation

Moderation is important with your temperatures, but also with your food quantities. When you find something that works, a meal you are able to eat with no issues, sometimes you may be so thrilled that you actually overeat. This can send you spiraling as well. Watch the quantities, and be sure to eat slowly, chewing each bite. This brings us back to mindfulness, and allowing enough time with our meals to be able to eat without rushing, and with care. **I am an adventurer, a risk-taker, a live-outside-the-box-er, but in the world of healing from IBS, moderation is key.**

Elimination Diets

As I mentioned in the Common Culprits section, there are some foods that are now recognized as common causes of symptoms for people with IBS: corn, gluten, wheat, eggs, dairy, yeast, peanuts, soy, and sugar. When I learned this, and how often these foods could be a cause of irritation for the gut, I decided to just eliminate them all, for a while, and see what happened. I did not really think that corn was an issue for me, but I eliminated it anyway, to be absolutely sure that I wasn't just kidding myself. I understand that this list may feel daunting, as you may already feel like you can't eat anything, but keep these two things in mind:

1. **Eliminating all of these foods is not intended to be for the rest of your life.** You get to set the (realistic) time frame, and you get to try to reintroduce them when you're feeling better, if you so choose.
2. **Believe me, once you start to feel better, the little bit of hardship eliminating these foods may have caused will be so worth knowing what you can safely tolerate in your diet going forward,** *you may likely forget the hardship altogether*.

Possibly more important than eliminating corn, wheat, eggs, dairy, yeast, peanuts and sugar from your diet is to consider removing all highly processed, ultra-refined foods from your diet. As a general rule, this refers to

1. anything that has a list of ingredients,
2. comes in a box or is packaged, or
3. is unrecognizable. This simply means, can you tell what it was when it grew in the ground? If not, it's unrecognizable and likely, it is highly processed and ultra refined.

The reason for this is that there are so many additives in foods that can cause irritation, upset, and imbalance that you may never have suspected. For example, I was innocently trusting that my unsweetened almond milk was "safe" and could not possibly be causing any issues. I never thought to check the ingredients list, because I thought surely it was just almonds, knowing that there was no sweetener added. Little did I know that gums, like xanthan or guar, are often used as a thickener, and come to find out, I was not tolerating those gums well at all (I can't even tell you what a "gum" is, let alone recognize it in its natural state!).

Another example of this for me was eating non-dairy ice cream for a while thinking I was just fine. It was non-dairy and sugar-free. In a pretty short amount of time, I discovered that the additives needed to create a palatable non-dairy ice cream that was also sugar free were not friendly at all to my digestion. Once again, the mysterious gums were present, as well as a variety of other unrecognizable ingredients. At first I thought I would go crazy from trying to track all those additives in everything I ate, and then I realized the easier path was to eliminate any processed, refined foods – even the ones that seemed "healthy" (dairy free, sugar free). I decided to set all those aside and just focus on whole foods, meaning,

1. foods in their natural state (usually no ingredients list needed)

2. foods typically not in a box (canned or frozen are okay), and

3. foods that are recognizable. This means, can you tell what it was when it grew in the ground? Is there anything about it that hints at what it may have been in its original, natural state? For example, dried fruits are pretty recognizable, so although they are processed (dehydrated), they likely do not have a long list of added ingredients and you can tell it was a berry or fruit by looking at it (recognize it). A muffin, on the other hand, will likely have many additives and a list of ingredients, and it may be very hard to tell what it was originally, when it grew in the earth (because it is a mish mash of processed ingredients).

There are different trains of thought on how long to eliminate these foods. Things to consider are how poorly you feel (how bad your symptoms are), and how long they have been that bad. The worse you feel and the longer you've felt that way can be a pretty good gauge of how much time you need to heal. Don't worry - having symptoms for years doesn't mean you have to eliminate these foods for an equally long period of time, but a good rule of thumb is three months to a year. I eliminated them for three months, along with processed foods, at the same time I was focused on a holistic approach to the other areas of my life, and that worked for me.

I feel it's important to point out that although I *can* tolerate processed foods now and don't have any issues with xanthum gum or other hidden ingredients, I still steer clear of them. I firmly believe that along with a few other notable reasons, those unrecognizable, highly processed, ultra-refined foods I call "carby carbs" are part of what got me into such a bad state in the first place, along with stress. I wasn't even eating that many - but I did grow up drinking coca-cola (high-fructose corn syrup), and certainly lots of breads, bagels, and other refined baked goods throughout my early years.

A very important distinction to make with any kind of elimination diet is that **you may find not only what you can tolerate as you heal, but that as you heal, you can tolerate more and more**. There is a significant difference between the two: one assumes that you will find something that you cannot tolerate, which implies "ever", and the second statement, the one I encourage you to be open to, is that **you may find that as your body heals, there are no foods you cannot tolerate.** Put another way, *you may find you can tolerate more foods after healing your gut than you could most of your life.* **It's entirely possible that as time goes on, and you get better and healthier and stronger, that there will be fewer and fewer foods that you find to be possible irritants or that cause a digestive issue.** Let me tell you, it's just a wonderful bonus to this journey back to health that I did not anticipate, and in fact, would never have believed possible. I would have been happy to just keep limiting my diet, avoiding dairy and processed foods if it meant I could feel normal. How wonderful it is that I continue to feel normal (well, in the sense of digesting normally, with no distress), and I can incorporate even more foods into my diet than I did prior to falling so horribly out of whack. My hope is that you are able to discover the same thing.

The FODMAP diet

Oh, I had such high hopes for the famed FODMAP diet. I even learned what the acronym stood for: Fermented Oligosaccharides, Disaccharides, Monosaccharides, and.... well, now I've forgotten, but no matter, because knowing what it stood for didn't really help me utilize it as a solution.

The FODMAP diet is a way to categorize foods based on the elements that they contain. It's not their vitamins and nutrients so much as their chemical composition. There are foods that are "high FODMAP", which mean you should steer clear if you have digestive issues, and there are foods that are considered low

FODMAP, which are deemed generally safe for folks with digestive issues, and some foods somewhere in between. I was introduced to the FODMAP diet some years ago when I had an attempted colonoscopy, and the doctor said, "Oh. You have IBS. Try the FODMAP diet." The only thing he told me about it was that I could eat anything on the FODMAP diet that was in the low-FODMAP category.

Welp. I found that was not exactly the case.

At the time I had been eating basically rice and kale, and a protein like chicken or ground turkey, and that was really the extent of my meals. I would have rice and turkey for breakfast, sometimes I could tolerate different things for lunch, and then dinner was usually something very safe (what I thought was safe) like the rice, kale, and a protein. So when he said you can eat anything on the low FODMAP diet in the low FODMAP category, I went for it. I mean, I really went for it. After such a restricted diet for so long, to have a doctor say I could eat the buffet was like being gifted freedom to the entire castle after being kept in a room with no window.

What I found is that there were things on the low FODMAP side that I shouldn't have switched to right away after eating such a limited diet. That was a big, huge lesson right there --- if you take nothing else from this book, please know that **radical changes in our diets are an issue even when our bodies are healthy and our digestive system is functioning normally.** When we are in the throes of a flare up or even just experiencing a not-healthy digestive process, making extreme changes like adding brand new foods, especially a lot of them over a short time, does not a good plan make. After some time, I learned that there are things on the low-FODMAP diet that I still won't eat, because they are highly processed and refined food that are just, generally speaking, unhealthy, and may cause inflammation or other pesky issues.

During this "You have IBS, eat FODMAP" adventure, I had an appointment with a dietician during the subsequent food festival, and we basically spent the entire appointment looking up labels on gluten-free pancakes. She's like, "You should be fine with gluten-free pancakes. You should be able to tolerate gluten-free pancakes", because, to her reasoning, they fall in the low-FODMAP category. The 45-minute appointment was spent with her Googling the labels of GF pancakes, and my hopes for help were dashed once again. And it's not really her fault - I think she just didn't understand IBS, and she didn't really understand the FODMAP diet. Just because a person is a dietician or nutritionist or medical doctor does not make them an expert in digestive health. It may seem strange, but it's true.

My experience with the dietician is not shared to rip on dieticians or to say that none of them know what they are doing. **My point is that you have to find what works for you, regardless of what the general consensus may be.** This is the second tenet of the Freedom Framework, and it holds true with our physical health, as well as other areas. Look, the American Dietetics Association does a great job providing us with information about how much protein the average person needs, how much salt is within reasonable limits for most people, how many vitamins and how much of them the general population needs, etc., but the reality is that we are all unique individuals, with different body sizes, different exercise routines, different health issues...so isn't it plausible that your needs may differ from the general population? Is it possible that just because something is gluten free and low FODMAP, you may not be able to tolerate it, for some other reason? This is not meant to discourage you from seeking medical or expert advice. On the contrary, *use all the professional input you have at your disposal!* **I encourage you only to remember that <u>you know you best</u>, and if something just doesn't add up, and doesn't fit your experience, <u>you get to make decisions about what you feel is best for you.</u>** Remember the medical practitioners who insisted that the no-added-sweetener carbonated seltzer water could not possibly be causing me to be bloated? When I stopped drinking it, the bloating stopped. So who is right? It doesn't matter! *I* get to choose to stop drinking it anyway, and ***they*** get to believe it could not have been related! **You do you**. I encourage you to take care of yourself in the ways that feel good and empowering to you.

There is a FODMAP app that lists nearly every food you can think of, in any variety of state (raw, cooked, prepared with condiments, boxed foods, etc.) and says whether they are definitively Safe, Be Careful, or Avoid. While I know that the FODMAP has helped many people, and that it is very scientifically based for categorizing foods, I do not find that the Safe foods align with what I found worked for me. This resulted in me (foolishly) eating a lot of the Safe FODMAP foods suddenly, and then regretting it greatly. A broad example of this are the insoluble fibers listed as Safe by FODMAP standards, but as an IBS participant, I found they are not always Safe and certainly not to begin a meal with.

Interestingly, I also did not find all the FODMAP Avoid foods to be unsafe for me, either. An excellent example of this are the beans and legumes. Beans have a reputation for causing flatulence (gas), and while this can be true for many people, it doesn't mean they are a digestive disrupter, necessarily. It just means you might pass gas as they move through your intestines. Beans are very often primarily soluble fiber, and therefore, became an excellent option for me. I have found that when using canned beans, rinsing them well before warming/eating them helps reduce the gas, and, I have found that since I have eliminated so many other digestive disruptors (breads, processed foods, carby carbs, etc.), I rarely have much gas, if any, even from beans. They are not only a great source of soluble fiber, but also are very nutritious.

Now, remember the rule about moderation here. Whenever we find something new that could work, we may tend to "overdo" - be sure to add them slowly to your diet, if you choose to give beans a try.

Think of it as a playdate with your intestines. They are just meeting beans perhaps for the first time or after a long hiatus. Plan just a short little get together to see how everyone gets along.

Another issue with the extensive FODMAP list was that often foods were Safe or Avoid depending on how they were prepared or what state they were in. For example, the FODMAP guide may say that soy in the form of a soybean is high FODMAP/Avoid, but that soy sauce is Low FODMAP/Safe[22]. Using the approach that worked for me, the Common Culprit list suggests that we steer clear of these foods in any form, until we are feeling quite well, consistently, and then reintroduce it, (for example, soy) in its various forms to see if it's an issue. There is nothing wrong with either approach, however I found that eliminating soy altogether, for a period of about three months, was far easier than trying to keep track of which soy was "good" and which was to be avoided.

I also believe the FODMAP diet isn't really a lifelong diet. It could be used to find out if certain chemical compositions are the cause of your issues (mine were not). That was a missing piece of information for me when I was trying out the FODMAP diet, and it may have served me better had I come at it from a "let's use this as a testing ground" tool instead of having a party with all the "Safe" foods, all at once.

The FODMAP categories have helped me, though, in other ways. Well into my recovery (perhaps a good year after feeling much better) I would still refer to the low FODMAP category sometimes just kind of as a double check. What's really amazing is now I can eat most of the foods, even in the high FODMAP category too. That too has evolved as my wellness has improved. There were some foods that took a long time for me to get to tolerating, and again, everyone is different, but some interesting ones that took a while for me to nail down were xanthan gums and guar gums,

---

[22] FODMAP categories may change over time. These examples were my experience at the time of writing this book.

which are oddly enough added to unsweetened almond milk. The less I ate foods with an ingredient list, the better I did (and still do). Multiple ingredients complicates things.

If you're interested in using the FODMAp to help you gauge your choices, there is a wonderful app you may find of interest called the MONASH FODMAP app. It's free, and very extensive. If you're interested in the foods that I found to be in contradiction to my soluble fiber/safe-for-IBS list, check out Appendix E in the back of this book.

To Track or Not to Track

Tracking your food and symptoms, no matter if it's via an app or a paper log, or notes to yourself, or texts to a coach, can feel like a full time job. If it revealed greatly helpful truths, insights that you couldn't get otherwise, I would say it would be worth it, but I did not find that to be the case.

Truth be told, I spent a lot of time tracking my symptoms in relation to specifically what I ate, devising complex logs and charts, downloading and familiarizing myself with apps for food and digestion, and exerting a lot of energy into comparing my food-symptom patterns, all without a great deal of success. I'm going to share with you the pros and cons of each effort so you can decide for yourself what is right for you.

One of the biggest pros of tracking my food and symptoms was that it made me very mindful of not only what I was eating, but also how I felt. I, a holistic wellness coach, thought I was being mindful and aware of what I ate, but tracking really helped me see some truths that I hadn't considered. **Tracking can also help you really notice how stress impacts you, how your emotions impact you, and how the emotions may be tied to your stress, and to your eating.** *Being truly mindful and aware is an important, if not one of the most important, first steps to gaining your health* *back.* That said, if the tracking becomes a source of stress, if it causes you anxiety or creates negative emotion, then there are other ways. Tracking is not a must, by any means, and does not have to go on endlessly either. You can use it for a while if it's working for you, and not continue if it becomes unuseful.

Tracking can also be useful when you start to introduce new foods, or reintroduce foods you had eliminated for a while.

Logs and planners

I tried using logs and planners for tracking that I found online, but felt that they did not allow for the detail that I wanted in relation to my experiencing symptoms very, very often. Remember that when things were very bad, once I had awoken the beast of my digestive process by consuming anything (even liquid), I was often a victim to my symptoms every fifteen minutes or so, for the first hour or even two, until it finally slowed to 20 minute increments, then 30, then once an hour, until we started over at lunch. I felt I needed to track the severity (frequency) of my symptoms, because there was always that odd day out, one morning every week or ten days, when I was not suffering to a great degree. Also, I tried keeping track of the kinds of symptoms, keeping copious notes about the pain level, and the stool quality. I was desperate to make sense of it all and find what I thought for sure was The Culprit or the several causes that would be the thing to turn me around. I do not now believe that you, or anyone, needs to focus (fixate) on your misery to that degree, especially knowing what I now do about the holistic picture and the smarter ways of grouping your foods to encourage healthy digestion.

I did create some logs, basically just a chart with the time of day in 15 minute increments on the left side, and the day itself across the top, split into two columns per date - one column for the food I ate and one column for the symptoms I experienced. I spend more time in the online course I've created on how to use the logs, if you so choose. Check out the Where to Go from Here section at the end of this book for more information about the online course and other resources available to you.

Apps

There are also several tracking apps available. One that I liked was the Cara Cares app. It is a free app that lets you track your food, an extensive list of symptoms (bloating, stomach pain, heartburn, constipation, etc.), your stool quality, your water intake, and your stress. The paid version gives you access to a registered dietitian via their Chat feature. You may find this app helpful on a varying scale - some may find it incredibly helpful, some may find it helpful to reveal some things you hadn't considered, and some may find it helpful as changes to your lifestyle (food intake, exercise, stress levels) are adjusted. Others may not find it helpful at all. Remember, you do you!

A Word about Over-the-Counter Options

I took over the counter bismuth (brand name: Pepto Bismol) for years. Then, I took the bismuth and a prescribed anti-anxiety medication each morning for years. It may or may not have helped, it may or may not have hurt, but I can tell you that when I stopped relying on the bismuth, and allowed my body to respond to foods, it took only a short time to see that I had probably been hindering the homeostasis by doing a hard brake, when a gradual slow down was possibly more what was needed. Consult with your trusted practitioner, but consider that the more "interrupters" you add, the harder it is again for your digestive system to find its own equilibrium. In my experience, and as I have said, moderation with over-the-counter quick fixes may also be key.

These are truths for everyone, but again, for those of us trying to heal a digestive issue, follow these simple rules and your body will thank you for it:

- Chew slowly.
- Take small bites.
- Eat moderate portions.
- Don't eat in a rush, or standing up if you can help it.
- You do not have to clear your plate. You don't have to heap on the food - you can get more if you're still hungry and feel you are tolerating well. You are in charge.

You can do this.

Your Wellness Lifestyle

As I hope I've been alluding to, there are a whole bunch of other things that come into play with your digestive health, besides food, which I collectively call your Wellness Lifestyle. Many of the following options have the significantly important added benefit of helping to reduce stress levels.

Downtime and Rest

A significant step in the right direction was simply, getting adequate rest. I found this did not mean necessarily just a good night's sleep. It meant really allowing downtime, allowing naps, allowing checking out and resting. Truly, fully, finding moments of rest for the sole purpose of selfcare. If someone had told my prior to dedicated-to-healing self to do this, I would have scoffed and declared I did not have the time, and that besides, I got enough sleep at night. Here is what I learned when I shed this view and my protests: *I needed a lot more rest, for a much longer period of time than I would have ever guessed, before I felt my body had finally gotten caught up/fully rested.* At the time I began to incorporate mindful downtime into my busy life, I can tell you that it seemed difficult and even problematic to try to find moments of quiet. For the many years prior to this new chapter of my life, I had never been able to benefit from meditation or even yoga, because I was on such a fast-paced "get 'er done" mindset that my monkey mind didn't quit the chatter, and I didn't work hard enough to rein in the chatter or to place enough importance on why I should. I was a single mother, yes, I worked three jobs at certain points, yes, but *all the more reason* to allow for rest, moments of de-stress, and downtime! Here's how I began to overcome the old, unhelpful habits of go-go-go and "I don't have time" and "it's not that important" excuses:

First, I just did little bits, little moments here and there. I started by pausing in the morning, before even lifting my head from the pillow, to just...take a moment. Breathe, and enjoy my breath. Sometimes, I would set an intention for the day, that might be as simple as "I will find another five minutes today to pause and just breathe". And I would.

As I became more accustomed to the quiet morning time, the goal to incorporate more time during the day became more prominent. I began to set a reminder on my phone for every hour, first with just the note, "Breathe", and then later, to other things I wanted to refocus my presence with, like "I am strong and healing", "I am doing very well", and many other combinations of self-encouragement to help me gain back control of my central intention, which was to get well.

I tried meditating again, here and there, and found it difficult for many, many months, so I just allowed the moments, little secret moments of quiet, inward focus upon my breath, upon something I was happy about or an image of beauty I recalled, sometimes sitting at my desk, perhaps in my car, perhaps between sessions and meetings and appointments or even between shifting to the next task. *Just a few moments began to make a world of difference.*

Then I started to take a few minutes during the middle of my day, at lunch, to just close my eyes. There is a wonderful app called Insight Timer that has not only traditional meditations, but also very thought-provoking speakers, and soothing music. The app lets you use their "Discover" option, and you can choose however much time you have and what you would like to participate in, so I would for example choose "5 minutes" and "music", and I would just close my eyes and listen. I began to be able to fall into deep relaxation during this time, and even though it was only 5 minutes,

I would re-emerge from this state refreshed, and noticeably calm and clear-headed. This occurred even before I had strong confidence that my belly wasn't going to send me running for a bathroom.

Then I started taking ten minutes. Easily. And looking forward to it.

The more I incorporated downtime and rest into my day, the more time I found I had to do so, and to actually *want* to. I began to take just ten minutes right after my work day ended as well, to lay my head back, close my eyes, and just listen to something pleasant and breathe before shifting into the next portion of my day. Ten minutes. It began to work wonders.

In addition to these newly instituted moments of calm, I walked. A lot. I have always been a walker, and my two dogs and I would regularly walk in the woods, sometimes for 20 minutes, and sometimes 1-2 hours. I found that after incorporating my new, quiet moments into my life, my walks became richer as well, and my thoughts, previously swirling and creating to-do lists and filled with anxious planning and action, formerly checking my phone, texting, taking calls while walking, instead became more present, and clearer, and calmer. The walks themselves did not change. *I* changed, and from that, the walks became even greater balms to my health. **This is the holistic nature of healing. When you make even small improvements in only one or two areas, it can have an exponentially improved impact into other areas.** The first tenet of the Freedom Framework says we are just shooting for the next best thing, and this is an excellent example of how that small little practice can have vastly profound results.

Many months later, in fact nearly a year after the point I became symptom free, I found I was not only able to meditate, but even enjoy it. It has become a regular practice for me as part of my healthy lifestyle, and though I don't do it for especially long periods, it has become a regular and wonderful part of my days, allowing me downtime, quieting of my mind, and connecting to the inner support that I have within me.

Healing Modalities I Tried

Before jumping into this next session, I just want to remind you that it's important to employ your "beginner's mind", and to be open to new possibilities. I share this information to give you "food for thought". If something resonates and your gut instinct is that it sounds useful, helpful, then listen to your gut! If it sounds like not the right thing for you, listen to that too - and remember that you can come back to that as an option another day if you choose. This is about creating the care you need, unique to beautifully and wonderfully unique you.

Hypnosis

Fortunately for me, I stumbled on some research that claimed hypnosis was proving useful for healing from IBS. I had experienced hypnosis a couple of other times in my life, and would not have said it was useful. Once, many years prior, I had tried to use it to quit smoking, and once, I was supposedly hypnotized at a party, except I was not. Nevertheless, I decided to try it again, in keeping with my being open to possibilities and to quieting the excuses, the ego that says "Been there, tried that". The results were interesting.

The first program I tried was a six-week, $100 app that I used diligently for 6 weeks. Though I did not see any immediate relationship between the daily sessions or alleviation of my symptoms, I did find that the dedication to doing the hypnosis for 6 weeks allowed me to prioritize some additional downtime into each day, which I no doubt benefited from. Shortly after the 6-week mediation, I came across a 100-day hypnosis for IBS, and decided to give that a try too. For whatever reason, I found this one a little more complicated, because there was a specific order to do the various sessions in (not consecutively), and I was very surprised by the sessions themselves, as they walked me down paths in my mind I had not visited before.

They were remarkably comforting, despite the unfamiliarity and the needing to stay organized around which session was due each day. These ranged from 30 minutes to perhaps an hour in length, and I found myself after only a week of daily sessions really looking forward to them. I can't say that I was truly hypnotized or if I simply fell asleep (which I did, often), so again, much needed rest may have been at play, but I did find myself recalling the imagery as I got through my still-rough mornings and sometimes unexpected bouts of anxiety (digestion-related or not). As I completed the 100 days, I was not "completely" healed, but I have no doubt the sessions helped me escalate the rate of my healing, due if nothing else to the very pleasant imagery, the mandatory down time, and the comfort that came with recalling the strength of the sessions available to me, at any given moment.

Often you may just need someone to prop you up a bit. To not feel so alone, and to believe in you. It's like having your own personal coach, as you groom the inner coach inside of you. (It's one of my favorite things about being a coach - helping to encourage as the person I'm supporting builds the foundations needed to support him or herself.) *You've got greatness inside of you. You have great strength and ability.* **Leaning on someone is not weakness. It is simply good self-care.** The hypnosis sessions helped me feel supported, even though they were just recordings I purchased. I felt I was treating myself well, taking good good care of myself. I found they were remarkably comforting in some rather unexplainable way.

Visceral Massage
Another very helpful addition to my healing journey were a couple of kinds of massage. I don't really mean going and getting a back or shoulder massage, for example, although that's wonderful. If it

reduces your stress, you should do it! But in addition to that kind of massage is the ability to do your own organ massage. I learned where my organs were inside my body and I spent time massaging my organs by massaging my abdominal area and, as woo-woo as it may sound, sending good intentions to my organs and appreciating my digestive system. Really getting to know it, in the sense of checking in, **listening inward to how my organs felt, and making them more of an ally instead of an enemy**. The shift from hating what was going on inside my body, to trying to make peace with it and figuring out what it needed from me, was significant. There's lots of YouTube videos out there for learning how to do what's called visceral manipulation or visceral massage or organ massage. Remembering that **our body is on our side** helps alleviate some of the resentment and frustration associated with long-term states of unwell.

Myofascial Release

I also stumbled on another option called myofascial release. I found out about this because I was looking for a practitioner who did visceral manipulation, before I learned how to do it myself (thanks, YouTube). I found a woman who was listed as offering visceral manipulation, but when I met with her, she shared that she also did what's called myofascial release. The myofacia is the webbing or the netting that is throughout all of our bodies and can hold tension, which can cause specifically our organs to be restricted in some ways. I don't pretend to be an expert on it by any means, but I can tell you that I found a great deal of relief from just a few sessions of that type of massage as well.

The Psoas Muscle

I do also go for "regular" massage whenever I am able, and one day, my massage therapist worked on my psoas muscle. I had read that a tight psoas muscle could impact digestion, and she was very familiar with what I was referring to. She informed me that a tight psoas muscle can interfere with blood flow and nerve impulses to the pelvic organs, interfering with digestion. Interestingly, it can also affect blood flow and nerve impulses to the legs, which may explain the odd leg and foot pain I experienced for a while that I mentioned in the Symptoms section. A tight psoas muscle can also interfere with the absorption of food by the gut. Mine was definitely tight, and after she worked on me, I felt yet more relief with my symptoms.

Colon hydrotherapy

Colon hydrotherapy is a technique for flushing the colon with water by a trained technician. The first time I had it done, it was terribly painful (remember those highly sensitive intestines that had been inflamed for so long), but I felt quite a lot better for days after. The second time I did it, about a year later, I did not have substantial improvement. So why do I mention it? I'm just offering you information. Remember, take from this book what resonates, and just let the rest go until or if you wish to revisit it again later.

Healing from IBS, from any illness of the body, heart, or mind, is so much more than just diet, or medicine, or any one singular thing. *It's the big picture that will make the difference in healing and wellness, in all areas of your life.* These are other areas that really contributed to my finding balance again with my digestive health, and ultimately in my overall wellness.

Supplements

Though you may be inclined to throw supplements and herbs and all sorts of remedies at this situation, keep in mind that the more new and different things you add, the harder it is for your body to trust what's coming and respond accordingly, the more challenging it becomes for you to sort out what's really having a negative impact. Just because something works for the general population does not mean that it will have the same effect on you, until your gut is calmer and can process the new addition somewhat normally.

Always check with your trusted health practitioner for support with your decisions.

I found two major exceptions to that general rule: the addition of a good quality probiotic. You cannot take a probiotic instead of eating well, instead of being attentive to your stress levels or your food choices or your sleep or those other things, but you *can* consider adding a probiotic on a consistent basis for a period of time as a strong and proven support for the gut. The ones I like are listed in the Where to Go from Here section and on my website.

The second is a product called Juice Plus that I was skeptical of at first. It is whole fruits and veggies in capsule, and while there are several options out there, Juice Plus really won me over with its high quality, all organic, highly researched product. It helped me really feel I was giving my body some good nutritional support. If you are concerned that you are not retaining the nutrients from your food, this product if nothing else can help set your mind at ease that you are at least providing additional nutritional value until you are well enough to get it from whole food sources. Many who take the product also report that it helps calm the digestive tract, perhaps thanks to the many thousands of phytonutrients. The company backs up its claims with tons of information and studies, all of which are available for you to read. I would again caution you to integrate these slowly, kindly, and gently, if you choose to try them. Learn more on the Where to Go from Here or my website.

Just for the sake of information, CBD is gaining in popularity for treating digestion issues[23], and I did try a rather expensive (supposedly high quality) gummy, but I did not notice any change. good or bad.

23

https://www.algeacare.com/de-en/medical-cannabis-treatment-of-irritable-bowel-syndrome/

Create a Wellness Team

Diagnosing IBS involves a number of tests, which, if you truly have IBS, often come back as negative, inconclusive, or not showing any abnormalities. If you've ever heard, "We didn't find anything," and especially if you've heard it many times, it can be not only frustrating, but also oddly disappointing, rather than relieving. Not because sufferers of IBS *want* something to be wrong. No indeed, our greatest fear is that something is radically wrong. But, we do want answers. When you hear that yet another test came up with no information, you may likely feel like yelling, "What do you mean? You didn't find *anything?* There's something so clearly not right!"

There is a lingering cloud of doubt that hangs over the sufferers of IBS, in that others don't necessarily understand or even accept the awfulness of the condition. I know I felt at times problematic, needy, embarrassed, defensive, and scared. It is very, very typical of IBS to not have a lot of "provable" evidence, because the disorder is diagnosed by ruling out other diseases, things that would show evidence of something like, say, an inflammatory response, or perhaps a visible lesion seen on an MRI. Very often, you have to go through a lot of tests to get an accurate IBS diagnosis, and very often, these tests are not only unpleasant, studies have shown they can be **more** uncomfortable and painful for people with IBS than people who do not have IBS[24]. This is significant, because you are then possibly at a place where your practitioners are doing due diligence by making sure, with absolute certainty, they have not missed any other possible culprit for your symptoms, but where you, enduring test after test, are in such pain sometimes, that chasing down yet another "possibility" can leave you feeling resentment toward your practitioners and really dread seeking further "care".

---

[24]

https://aboutibs.org/treatment/understanding-and-managing-pain-in-ibs/

The important take-away here is not be fearful of the tests. It is to recognize that certainly your practitioners can lose sight of the lived experience of the person (you) enduring the tests. I am not by any means suggesting you forgo testing. That is a personal decision each person must make, for each test, and each step of your journey. I am suggesting that you consider that your practitioner may need some reminding of just how painful some tests can be. When your intestines are so inflamed, normal procedures that don't hurt others can be a whole different ball game for sufferers of IBS. There are steps that can sometimes be taken to help ease the pain, so it's worth discussing.

In the world of alternative medicine, there are some pros and cons to understand as well. Often, in my experience anyway, I found that my naturopath (N.D.) (a medically trained doctor of naturopathy, the use of plants and herbs) had a much broader ability to conduct tests than my nurse practitioner (N.P.) (Western traditional medical care). My nurse practitioner was often either not able to order certain tests for me, or she was not even aware some tests existed. For example, with the N.D., I was able to have my stool analyzed for a wide variety of bacteria and parasites, which certainly helped to again rule those out as possible culprits, which is important. The methods for approaching a parasitic infection are different from the approach to IBS. The naturopath was also able to review the medical tests done by the Western medical team, which helped inform her of other possibilities. She also noticed a very low ferritin on my blood work that was missed by my nurse practitioner, and which I was able to address. It may or may not have been related to the IBS - my point is that I found having the support of the naturopath (alternative medicine), in addition to my nurse practitioner (traditional medicine), helped me feel more empowered. **The more people you have on your side, who are caring for you in ways that feel like support, the better for you!**

Your wellness team can include whomever you feel supports you.
**It can be family, friends, a digestive coach or holistic coach like
me, and even people online who may understand what you are
going through.** There are a number of groups on Facebook for
example that provide information and the ability to connect with
others who may be experiencing similar things. Be aware, though,
that I found many times the negativity in these groups was not
helpful, even harmful. It was sometimes very hard to believe I
would become well when seeing post after post of misery, with no
answers, and no relief. There is nothing wrong with sharing how
hard this is, how hard it is to live with this sometimes, and to look
to others for comfort and understanding. However, if the posts are
bringing you down, taking the wind out of your sails, or otherwise
bringing negativity into your world, consider finding other options.

Nature

Oh nature. What a lovely, lovely gift nature is. *Being in nature
and perceiving its magic, tiny little miracles happening all the
time, can really help pull you out of your head and away from
your anxiety and the noise of your mind, if you allow it.* I am an
avid nature lover, but if you are not, that does not mean that nature
doesn't help you in other ways.

Experiencing nature, or even watching videos of beautiful nature
scenes, can reduce negative feelings such as anger, fear, and stress.
Exposure to nature can induce pleasurable feelings and make you
feel better emotionally by reducing blood pressure, lowering your
heart rate, reducing muscle tension, and lowering the production of
stress hormones.[25]

---

[25]
https://www.takingcharge.csh.umn.edu/how-does-nature-impact-our-wellbe
ing#:~:text=Being%20in%20nature%2C%20or%20even,the%20production
%20of%20stress%20hormones.

Here are ways I incorporate nature into my world on a regular basis:

★ Go for walks outside
★ Ride my bike
★ Sit on the stoop and feel the breeze
★ Listen to the birds chirping outside my window
★ Listen to the wind howl
★ Watch the snow swirl
★ Feel the heat of the pavement radiating up on to my skin
★ Notice the rustle of the leaves
★ Smell the dirt scent rising up from the earth
★ Hold a cool stone in my hand
★ Gaze at photos of nature, or take pictures of the natural world (visit my photo gallery for inspiration!)
★ Marvel at a tiny flower growing up through the cracks of a sidewalk

Whatever way you choose to incorporate nature into your world, I hope you do. I invite you to sign up for my Monday Mindset videos, a year's worth of one-minute videos of nature,, to help you find one minute a week to quiet your mind and open your heart, as my gift to you. Join the Monday Mindset email series by visiting the Where to Go from Here section at the end of this book.

I also have a gallery of natural photography you are welcome to peruse. You can order prints, mugs, pillows, phone cases, and more fun items to keep nature around you all the time. I donate a percentage of the profits to non-profits that support our natural world, so your purchase helps nature, while nature helps you! Check out the gallery at live-true-pixels.com.

Stretching and Strengthening

Although I have always thought of myself as active, riding my bicycle in my younger years as my preferred mode of transportation, and walking daily with my dogs for several decades, during those really awful years I became less and less mobile without even realizing it. I was so fearful of having an emergency moment, so turned inward to my bodily functions, without really being conscious of it, I became actually physically curved inward too, as though always a little hunched, a little rounded to protect my abdomen. I was, frankly, in a lot of pain too, a lot of the time, and not as apt to exert muscular tension, particularly in my core, which I found became soft and, well, weak. A weak core is not a good thing - our core muscles (the ones that wrap our abdomen around to the back) support our organs, our back, our posture, and provide stability and balance. I only realized how much I had lost once I began to feel better. I believe had I placed more intentional focus on gentle, small movements of my body, particularly for my core muscles that cradle, protect, and support my digestive organs, I may not have had the extreme amounts of pain I ended up with. I will never know if it's true, but I can tell you that I am certain that by providing more support and strength for my abdomen, I directly supported and strengthened my digestive system as a whole. Here are some gentle, small movements to consider incorporating into your life, **after checking with your trusted health practitioners** of course:

- Try to take regular walks, even if they are slow-paced and rather meander-y. Moving your body out in the world is a great way to "get out of your head" and just allow your body to do its thing.
- Add stretching to your days. Start with a few times a week, if it's difficult, then move up to daily. This does not have to be a full-on yoga practice. Simply laying on the floor

on your back, and pulling your knees to your chest can be a wonderful, gentle stretch that massages the organs.

- Go to YouTube for ideas for stretching to aid in digestion. There are several wonderful go-to floor positions I do on a regular basis. That's key - try to incorporate them into your life. This is not a one-and-done, or something to do only when you feel poorly. Make this part of your health routine.

- If you find that your core, your abdomen, has become weaker, or feel you may be "guarding" it by not using those muscles much, even tiny micro movements can help us regain that strength for stability and support. Again, YouTube is your friend for this.

- A really great, easy, and fun move is to simply stand with your feet in a position that feels stable to you, as you gently and slowly twist side to side at the waist, with your arms extended to the side of you, hands floating in the breeze. Like you used to when you were little, and waiting in a line somewhere. You are doing a slight spinal twist here, so again check with your trusted practitioner if you have concerns, but what you are also doing, importantly, is massaging your organs. Twisting is phenomenal for your digestion, and can help release stress in your belly area.

Establish a Routine of Self-Care

If your days are chaotic, and unpredictable, it does add another level of complexity to managing your symptoms and finding your way out of them. Some sense of normalcy, knowing basically what to expect for your day, and being able to plan your meals is a super helpful but not always possible piece of your success. It doesn't mean you can't get there, though - it just means you have to be creative about what you can control, and what you do know.

The more you can plan ahead, the easier your choices will be.
If your week continually gets away from you, despite your best
intentions, and you end up eating fast food or things you know are
no good for your gut, try to get ahead of that by meal planning at
least a few meals and grocery shopping during the weekend. If you
do fine grocery shopping, but regularly run out of time or energy or
desire to actually make the meals once your week is in full swing,
consider meal prepping on Sunday evening: chop some veggies,
marinate some protein - even cook things ahead of time if that will
help! You can even buy pre-chopped vegetables or pre-cooked
items (canned veggies for example just need to be heated). There
are so many ways this can look, and be a success. You do not have
to plan, prep, and cook every meal at the time of the meal in order
to be taking good care of your gut and your health. *The very best*
method is the one that brings you the most ease, and the greatest
sense of calm in your days. If you just can't see a way to make
meal planning and preparation easier, get support! The Where to
Go from Here section has some options for you..

Another good habit to establish is to have a back-up plan. Carry
snacks in your car if you think you might be running late, or get
stuck somewhere unplanned. Spend a little time perusing the
take-out menus of places in your world that will have some safe,
healthy options for you - even if you order all "sides" or appetizers,
if those are what work for you, that's absolutely acceptable and
that's good self-care! Another "plan ahead" trick is to always look
at a menu before you sit down at the restaurant, so you can take
your time plotting out the best order for your best gut care.

One thing for certain is that you will at some point, start your day
after a period of sleep. If you work nights, perhaps your day
doesn't start until afternoon for the rest of the world, but for you,
that's your morning. If nothing else, we all have a period of sleep
from which we awaken, and begin anew. This is a wonderful time
to establish not only some sense of routine and calm, but to really
set the tone for the day, regardless of what may come along.

Everyone's morning routines, or rituals if you like that term better, may look different. Mine evolve, and yours likely will as well (the third tenet of the Freedom Framework). Here are some ideas to consider incorporating into your morning, to help you find the surest footing to head out into the world:

- Before you lift your head from the pillow, think of something you really felt good about from the day before. If you can think of three things, great, but even spending time reliving that good feeling from just one small thing can really help your central nervous system stabilize.
- Set an intention for the day that supports you, lifts you up, recognizes your efforts at taking care of yourself, and makes you feel good. This can take as long or as short as you like, depending on how you do it. You can couple it with your gratitude moment, or you can take the time to journal about it, or you can repeat an affirmation as you rise from bed or shower. However you do it, really sink it into your mind.
- Place importance on your self-care first, before you do anything that can detract from that focus. This means, even if you must feed the dogs, make the morning beverage, perhaps get the children up, you can still "start" with a moment of setting your intention for the day. For example, I write in a little notebook each morning. I do it after I've let the dogs out, fed them, given them their medicine, tossed treats to the kitties to bat around, and have at least half a cup of warm beverage in me. I do not, however, look at my phone before doing this. I do not check my to-do-list or think unduly hard about anything my day holds. I do not hold silent angry conversations in my head in anticipation of an argument I may think could occur. I simply let that good-feeling memory from the day before carry me through these handful of chores, until I can sit down with my journal and the rest of my warm

beverage, and at the very least, set a nice intention for my day, such as "I will find humor in whatever comes my way today" or "I am strong, capable, and kind to myself" or "I am healing, and making the best choice available to me at any given moment for my continued health, physical, mental, emotional and spiritual". The idea here is not to hold yourself to an impossible standard, but to intend to do well by yourself and your goals, and to just do your best as you go through your day.

I like to revisit the previous day's journal entry as well, to remind myself of what felt good to me then. In this way, I am always building on my good feelings, day after day.

You may wish to incorporate some stretches into your morning routine as well. A really nice way to not let the day get away from you before you can get to your stretches is to **do them while you are still in bed**. There is no rule that says we must get on the floor in our leggings and hair in a ponytail. If you have some floor stretches, you can certainly roll out the yoga mat right next to your bed and make it part of a lovely morning ritual where you give your body the devotion it deserves.

If you have the time, perhaps try incorporating some meditation if that is up your alley, or some yoga. You may want to go for a walk around the block, breathing in the crisp morning air, listening to the sounds as the world awakens with you. If you don't have the time for these things, that's okay! It's not worth stressing yourself out, trying to fit in things that are intended to de-stress. And, you can always try to incorporate these into your routine later in the day, if that works better. The key is to make these things work for you, not against you, to add to your wellbeing, not detract from it.

Establishing routine, particularly at the beginning of your day, has the possibility to help you begin your day on solid footing, which can help manage your stress throughout the day even if symptoms go haywire later. A routine can keep you mindful of your ultimate goal as you move through your day. **Remember that it takes *practice* to establish these healthy routines;** if you do it for a couple of days, and then forget or get too busy for a couple of days**, just try again! There is no "failure".** *You get to just keep going. Tomorrow is a new day! Try again!* Better yet, when you realize at lunch you forgot to set your intention or take a moment finding something wonderful from the day before, do it then! *If the day has gotten away from you, take a few minutes to just breathe, wonderful deep breaths.* **This is your story. You get to write it in whatever way serves you best.**

What Works Will Change: True Freedom

I've mentioned the Freedom Framework here a few times and the basic tenets of it again are:

1. Striving for the next better [emotion, food, thought, experience, relationship, job, home]
2. Embracing what is unique to YOU, and understanding WHY
3. Mastering continued growth!(or, what is right for you in the moment will inevitably change as you continue to evolve, and as life continues to shift!)

I give you these as gifts to ease your burden as you find your way through this journey to wellness. The first gift allows you to just do your best, do what you can in the moment, to find what makes you feel just a little better, whether physically, mentally, emotionally, or spiritually. In terms of your IBS, this could look like trying to keep track of every morsel but recognizing that tracking your food to that degree is exhausting and only makes you feel worse, so this first gift lets you just stop doing that, for a while or until you feel inspired to try it again. **Things that are heavy and dragging you down get to be changed. Thoughts that feel defeating or emotions that make you want to just curl up into a ball, those are important to notice - so you can find a thought that feels just a little better** (from "I'll never get to well" to "I really want to get well" to "I am ready to make changes to help me get well"), **an emotion that feels slightly less heavy** (from fear of never getting well to a desire to get well, from a desire to get well to cultivating the courage to take the necessary steps).

The second gift is hopefully what I've been encouraging you toward - I can give you the information that I discovered in my journey, and I can tell you what worked for me, but **your journey may look different.** *None of us are the same.* If a specific diet worked for all of us, for health, wouldn't the whole world do it? The truth is we are all unique and there is much more to wellness than a formula-based program. I leave a lot in here for you to determine, and for some people, that is really frustrating. I cannot tell you exactly what you must do - but I absolutely believe you can find your way, and I hope what I've offered in this book helps inform you as you walk this path. If you determine that you want more support, be sure to check out my information on courses and coaching.

The third gift doesn't feel much like a gift at all, at first. **What you find works for you today will likely be different than what you find works not too far down the road.** *This is a good thing! This is life, life happening - if we found the one thing, one way, one diet, one routine, one path that "worked", then how are we growing?* What happens when something different occurs in our world, like a vacation, a job change, a loved one becomes ill, someone gets married, etc? **We need to adapt and flow with life as it happens for us. It is not happening** *in spite of* **our best efforts. The changes that occur** *are* **life happening.** Knowing that we have the tools at the ready to deal with changes can bring back a whole lot of joy and appreciation for the unknowns in our worlds, instead of resentment because we feel out of control or trepidation because we don't know what to do. **Learning to look forward to growth, and the changes that growth brings, helps us not only feel better equipped, but be better equipped to navigate the roads of our lives. How cool is that?**

There is an underlying but very important gift for you in all of this, whether anything I've said before this resonates or not, and that is:

There is no failure, no going backward, no keeping score, no guilt, and no shame

You get to be kind to yourself. You get to look at what you attempted and call it good. You get to have successes, and to celebrate each one. I see over and over this mentality of "starting over on Day One" if someone feels they have backslid, or missed a day of exercise, or had a bad morning after a couple good ones, and I say "NOT TRUE!"! You can't possibly be starting over on Day 1 or falling two steps back because you know more today! You know more today than yesterday and you know more right now than an hour ago and you are always moving forward with your journey. It may feel like a mountain, but you have not slid back at all. **You are always making progress in one way or another, and** *as long as you are being kind to yourself and trying your best to feel better, you are succeeding.* **The better you get at that piece, the faster the rest will follow.**

How can you manage these unexpected things? By expecting them! In terms of caring for yourself as you heal from IBS, if you have the food you need for the day planned out, anticipate what could occur that would make that plan need to be altered. Maybe you shopped on Sunday for the week, and plan to take your food with you in an insulated lunch box each day, but one day you forget your cooler. What could you do? Have some snacks on hand that you know you can tolerate, for one. Keep them in your desk drawer, your locker, your car. Make it a game, keeping ahead of the possibilities, and when the inevitable happens that you haven't anticipated, and you're left having to come up with something on the fly, try to seek out the excitement in it, versus the worry and anxiety. It could end up revealing something to you that you've been wanting!

Stay Diligent and Stay Strong

Another thing I noticed was that as I began to feel better, or even in those small windows when things felt calmer, I would gain such hope and confidence, and be so ravenously hungry, I would overeat, or eat fast, or eat too much and too fast, or eat too much variety, and too much of it. These are all things to consider and to do better than I did - try to keep yourself on a short leash until you can be sure you're really on the other side of the wellness balance, and not just caving into a moment of respite.

You will learn what is normal for you, and you will learn what your body's way of maintaining balance is and what works for you. We're all different. I don't think there's any one diet for any of us, but the exciting part is, is that you're so on your way. You are on your way to figuring out what works for you.

Pick Your Battles

I just also want to say a quick word about the "but"s and "what about"s perhaps going through your mind. But what about organic versus non-organic? What about local versus organic? Should I buy grain-fed versus organic meat? Should I become vegetarian? What if I am vegan? Maybe you are trying to lose weight, or worrying about gaining weight, or maybe you are already scarily underweight and concerned about losing more. Use your Wellness Team! Confer with your professionals! Lean on others!

Consider that there are two ways of looking at really any decision. There is a good side (the pros) and a not so good side (the cons). If you're living in an area where your organic produce has to come from a long distance away, then it's traveling on a truck for hundreds of miles and it's essentially dying the whole time that it's on the truck. More nutrients are available the sooner we eat freshly harvested produce. So is "fresher" better than "chemical/pesticide-herbicide-free"? We could spend many many days trying to make that determination, and to what end? Isn't your goal to feel better, in the easiest, quickest, calmest, kindest method available to you? Pick that one. The one that feels easy, calm, and kind, and gets you feeling better. Change it later if you wish. This is your life, for you to live how you choose.

Not too long ago I had one of these "but what about" moments. This was well into many months of feeling wonderful and not experiencing any symptoms of IBS. I had decided to start an herbal protocol to support my immune system that I was so excited about. I wanted to do it because my body has been so good to me, really, over all these years, taking me on so many adventures (the good kinds), and as I creep up in years, this protocol looked like just the gift I could give to my body. It involved 90 days of a pretty hefty vitamin, mineral, and herbal routine that had been suggested to me by my N.D., who is well aware of my digestive journey. I carefully eased into it, adding the new supplements little by little, until gradually, over 2-3 weeks, I was consuming the mega-doses this routine called for, and committed to sticking with it for the 90 days. About six weeks in, however, I realized I had been having more urgent bathroom needs, and what really awoke my attention was waking up each morning with my belly moaning like a ship going down. I immediately realized it was the mega-doses, and had to make a decision: should I continue, just power through, though my gut was clearly being negatively impacted? Or, should I stop the herbal routine completely? But what about wanting to support my immune system? I chose to stop completely for a week, to see if that was the cause, and sure enough, everything settled back to normal. I decided instead of the mega doses for the remaining days of the three-month routine, I would just do normal doses, and give my body that gift. It's a compromise. It's a personal choice. And those kinds of things will keep happening - new possibilities will arise and you'll have to choose what matters most to you as you move through your life. Choice is a wonderful thing.

Twisting yourself into knots and getting really stressed out about your choices won't help get you where you wish to be. **Take a step back and look at what feels the lightest to you. What feels the easiest in terms of your stress levels? What is your most immediate goal? To feel better. You can shift your focus to other concerns once you achieve this win, and think how good you'll feel doing it.**

The Truth of It

When I first started writing this book, I was about 6 months into my healing, and I felt on top of the world. Another 6 months after, and I felt even better. My new levels of wellness continued for a good two years, each one seeming like I was as healed and feeling as good as I could possibly feel, only to realize some months down the road, I was even better still. Does this mean it will take you years to feel better? Nope, that's not what I'm saying at all. What I am saying is that it took me years to feel as bad as I did to finally take the reins and make change, and I believe because I was so unwell for so long, my journey back to health took a while too. The good news is that it's not an eye for an eye - I felt unwell, in a state of experiencing IBS symptoms of some form or another since I was about 12 years old (in the 70s), growing increasingly worse in my 20s (in the 80s-90s), a gradual yet constant decline through my 30s and 40s, until finally I hit the breaking point, which became my ultimate turning point. So three years of a journey back to ultimate health after decades of unwell does not a long journey make! **I suspect if I had started paying closer attention earlier, had the tools and knowledge and resources I do now, I would not have declined to the degree I did, nor would it have taken as long to get better again.** *The sooner you can turn the tide, the sooner you can start living a full and healthy life again.*

Have you ever thought about people (myself included, perhaps you!) who consume too much alcohol for the feel-good-in the-moment, knowing they will experience the worst hangover the next day? I know a lot of people with IBS or other digestive limitations who decide to eat something they know they can't tolerate, because it sounds good and they aren't feeling strong or diligent or committed at the time. The general refrain is "F**k it,

I'm eating this." Enough of that attitude will only exacerbate the IBS symptoms into a new refrain of "I'm never eating that ever ever ever again" (much like, "I'm never drinking tequila again"). Funny what we humans do to ourselves, isn't it?

I somewhat prolonged my eventual crossing of the finish line to total wellness, because I would start to feel so much better, and celebrate with a rotten choice that would set me back again, sometimes for weeks. This was not necessarily alcohol. Perhaps it was a piece of pizza, or cake, or a very spicy food which I love, but which my gut was not yet ready for. **This was perhaps the hardest thing - staying the course, staying strong, sticking with my disciplined choices even once I was feeling really good.** The longer I stayed on the food choices that worked for me and didn't introduce things in the wrong order or try something new or otherwise muck things up, the longer the feeling well lasted. Those "new" moments of feeling well are such a gift, and they were the hardest moments through which to refrain from celebrating with something that pulled me back down again.

We are human, after all, and sometimes, a little "cheat" here or there is too good to pass up. My two cents on that is, never, ever cheat more than once a week as you are healing (and that means one food or beverage option, not one day of cheating), until you are really feeling so far out of the woods that you cannot even see them anymore, and can safely tolerate your choices normally again. You want to get well into the wellness, well beyond the unwell.

Depending on where you are in your journey, even once a week is playing with fire, but at the very least, just not more than that. Do that for yourself. Eventually, in not too long at all, you may find you are happily not having to consider any of those food choices "cheating" at all. The goal is to get there, and if it means a couple more months of steering clear, isn't that worth it?!

Another truth here is that **even healthy people with normal digestion sometimes have bad days!** One bad moment, a morning of unexpected diarrhea, or an occasional gurgling gut after a meal out does not mean your IBS is coming back full force! Nor does it even necessarily mean it's IBS, if you are truly out of the woods when it happens. I used to have that fear (good old anxiety) grip me when I had a rare moment like that, because it catapulted me back to when things were such a living hell, but the truth is that sometimes, we may just have a bout of unwelcome bacteria, or something else unexplained. Keep your cool, trust that you are treating yourself in the best way you can, doing your best, and trust that this will pass. If it continues, look honestly at your food choices, your lifestyle, your stress levels, and see if perhaps there is something you have incorporated that is not serving you. Are carby carbs sneaking their way into your diet? Maybe it's just not time for that. Have you been pushing yourself at work, or stressing out about something else in your life? Shift back to self-care as the primary focus, and see if that settles things down again. **This is a continual, lifelong process, *for everyone of us*, regardless of IBS or other functional disorders or any state of wellness. We are here to support our bodies as our bodies support us. This *is* what self care looks like.**

I know it's a bummer that you are going through this. I know it just sucks that you have this issue, when it seems that others can eat just about anything. When you are feeling low, like you won't make it out of this, or that you just don't have it in you to keep going, consider these truths:

- It may take longer than you like to feel better, but <u>it won't take as long as if you don't ever start.</u>
- **Sleep as much as you can, as much as your body needs.** Listen to your body, and *make sleep as important for your body as if you were a newborn.*
- **The very last thing to "heal" and for me, and it still sometimes rears its head, is the anxiety and stress around my digestion acting up.** Even now, years into my wellness, into my "no-longer-having-IBS", I will sometimes have that mental preoccupation and fear around an event, or an outing, wondering and worrying what the bathroom situation will be. For some of us, IBS has been rather traumatizing, so be kind to yourself about it, recognize the anxiety for what it is - a residual effect that you can allow to pass - and then, do that. Allow it to pass.
- **Be kind to yourself. Treat yourself as if you like yourself. Treat your body as if it is on your side,** *because it is.* It's doing its best to get back into alignment too, even if it feels like it is betraying you. **You and your body are a team.** Get to where you want to do good things for your body, like you do for a new friend. Ask your body what it needs, and listen.
- **Make friends with your organs.** *They are not your enemies.* Your lovely stomach, your amazing intestines, your oh so wonderful colon. **When you embrace your organs as being on the same side as you, as being in it together, it shifts some of that angry frustrated energy into a gentler, more empowered and calmer place from which to learn to truly listen to your gut.**

Where to Go from Here

Life is a journey, and yours happened to include a side adventure into the Land of IBS. The great thing is that you now see avenues and pathways that could lead you out of that muck, and onto greener pastures. It does take diligence, it does take determination, will power, strength, and even courage. I believe you have it in you, to make change that brings you to a better feeling place. And I'm here to help!

Visit www.lisathorne.me to:

- Book individual coaching sessions: Whether related to your IBS or something else, you are welcome to book sessions with me if you'd like one-on-one support.
- Check out my Favorite Products page for things that really helped me
- Sign up for my Monday Mindset emails, a nifty 60-second-or-less video of nature and a little write-up every Monday for a year, to bring one minute of calm and mindfulness into your week
- Get on the Freedom from IBS email list and get answers to the top ten questions I get about IBS, and to stay informed of courses, and more!
- Access the Freedom from IBS online course
- Peruse the photo gallery of nature and all its wonders (on the About page) o help incorporate some beauty, peace, and calm into your daily!
- Connect with me on the socials! (And reach out! I'd love to hear from you!)

No matter where you are in your journey, you're here now. It's as good a place to start as any! Remember that your goal is to feel well, and let your heart and, yes, your gut, lead you!

Appendix A: What I Drink When I Do a Gut Reset

Visit My Favorite Products page at lisathorne.me for links

Bone broth
-Check the ingredient lists (the fewer the items, the cleaner). I like the ones with high protein. Chicken seems to usually have the highest protein that I find.

Water

Water with a dash of fresh lemon juice can be very refreshing. If you don't have fresh, check out one I like that is bottled

Tea

-herbal, such as mint. Click the link on my favorite products for my favorite peppermint tea
-black or green - watch the caffeine!

Rice water:

1 C basmati or long-grain white rice
10 Cups water

Bring to a boil, then let simmer for 20 minutes
Strain out the rice, keeping the water
Let cool, then store in the refrigerator until use. Can be reheated for drinking.

Appendix B: Fiber Food List

Soluble Fiber - these are often root veggies (the part we eat grows in the ground) but can also be some fruits like bananas and plantains. They are "carbs" but not like ultra-refined, processed carbs.

- Potatoes, baked/mashed
- Beets
- Squash (acorn, butternut, pumpkin, etc.)
- Eggplant
- Banana
- Plantains
- Sweet potato
- Beans (also a protein)
- Lentils
- Chickpeas
- White rice
- Oats cooked well (start slow)
- Non-whole grain pastas

Insoluble Fiber - Often they are leafy, dark green, and have veins or are "stringy". They may have tough skins or peels, which are very insoluble.
- Spinach
- Kale
- Cabbage
- Onion
- Asparagus
- Broccoli
- Brussel sprouts
- Cauliflower
- Bell pepper

Both Soluble and Insoluble Fiber foods - Some (many) foods have both kinds of fiber. The soluble fiber foods usually have insoluble fiber in their skins, peels, and seeds.

- Potatoes (though the skin is not super insoluble)
- Eggplant (the skin is VERY insoluble)
- Tomato (watch the seeds and skin!)
- Zucchini (the insides of zukes are technically insoluble, but are usually well tolerated for IBS - remove seeds and peel just to be sure)

Appendix C: Healthy Fats & Beverages

Healthy fats:
These are fats that occur naturally in foods, or that are extracted from foods and not highly processed or modified. The best rule of thumb is to try never to eat fats first (even healthy ones). The best rule of thumb is to eat **soluble fiber first**, every time you introduce food into your body.

- Walnuts, pistachios, almonds, cashews, macadamia nuts
- Almond butter, peanut butter (watch the sugar content)
- Avocados
- Coconut
- Olives
- Oils from any of the foods listed here
- Pesto (it often has dairy, so check the ingredients if you are not doing well with dairy!)
- Olive-oil based mayo (if you know you tolerate eggs well)

Beverages
These beverages are almost always soothing, and safe for IBS:

- Peppermint tea, warm or cool
- Any herbal tea
- Bone broth
- Rice water
- Water, with a spritz of lemon juice
- Water infused with vegetables such as cucumber, melon, or blueberries (if you don't eat the produce, the infused water will not be a GI stimulant)

These beverages are considered GI stimulants or irritants, and not considered safe for IBS:

- Coffee
- Alcohol
- Soda, Pop
- Sugary Drinks
- High-fat drinks like coconut milk, dairy

Appendix D - A Guide to What I Felt Safe Eating, Depending on How I Was Physically Feeling

When my digestio n is consiste ntly… ...I felt comforta ble with these foods	☹	☹	😐	🙂	
Rice	Yes	Yes	Yes	Yes	Yes
Banana	Yes	Yes	Yes	Yes	Yes
Whole Wheat Toast	Nope	Nope	Nope	Nope	Nope
Kale	Nope	Nope	Yes, in moderat ion	Yes	Yes
Oatmeal, cooked	Yes, plain	Yes, plain	Yes, without a lot of "extras"	Yes, in moderat ion with added toppings	Yes, in moderation with added toppings until you

					know for sure
Potatoes, baked	Yes, plain	Yes, plain or with a little olive oil	Yes, without a lot of "loaded" extras	Yes, in moderation with the toppings	Yes, in moderation with a variety of toppings until you know for sure
Beets, cooked	Yes	Yes	Yes	yes	Yes
Carrots, cooked	Yes	Yes	Yes	Yes	Yes
Lettuce	Nope	Nope	Nope	In moderation, starting with a soluble fiber bite first	Yes
Spinach	Nope	Nope	cooked well	Cooked well or in moderation with a soluble fiber first, if raw	Yes
Eggplant	Nope	Yes, with no peel	Yes, with no peel	yes, even with	Yes, with or without peel

				peel	
Cold Coconut milk	Nope	Nope	Nope	Maybe with a smoothie with soluble fiber (bananas and blueberries) in the afternoon	Yes, but pay attention to first-thing-in-the am! I still do not do super cold first thing!
Blueberries	Nope	Nope	Yes, in moderation with other SF	Yes, in moderation	Yes
Beans and legumes (pinto, great northern, black, lentil)	Nope	Yes, cooked well	Yes, cooked well	Yes	Yes
Corn	Nope	Nope	Nope	As a test run	Yes (if the test run went well)
Soy	Nope	Nope	Nope	As a test run	Yes (if the test run went well)
Eggs	Nope	Nope	Nope	As a test	Yes (if the

				run	test run went well)
Dairy	Nope	Nope	Nope	As a test run	Yes (if the test run went well)
Yeast	Nope	Nope	Nope	As a test run	Yes (if the test run went well)
Peanuts	Nope	Nope	Nope	As a test run	Yes (if the test run went well)
Sugar	Nope	Nope	Nope	As a test run	Yes (if the test run went well)

Appendix E: Soluble Fiber versus FODMAP

The FODMAP diet lists nearly every food you can think of, in any variety of state (raw, cooked, prepared with condiments, boxed foods, etc.) and says whether they are definitively Safe, Be Careful, or Avoid. While I know that the FODMAP has helped many people, and that it is very scientifically based for categorizing foods, I do not find the "Safe" foods to align with what I found worked for me. This resulted in me (foolishly) eating a lot of the Safe FODMAP foods suddenly, and then regretting it greatly. The chart below compares some foods from the FODMAP diet marked Safe that conflict with the approach I use.

How to use this chart:

The "yes" in the first column indicates they are considered SAFE by FODMAP categorization.

The "yes" in the second column indicates these foods are **primarily soluble fiber**, and therefore not typically a gastrocolic trigger, and therefore safe in my experience as well. **If both of the first two columns say "yes", it is likely a very safe bet, even when you are feeling very, very frowny-faced about your symptoms**.

A "yes" in the third column indicates the food is **not primarily soluble fiber**, and according to what I found worked for me, a food I would avoid until feeling better (see chart above). **If there is a "yes" in the FIRST column and the THIRD column, there is a clash of approaches (FODMAP vs Soluble Fiber/what worked for me)**.

The fourth column indicates these foods are **high in FODMAPs and should be AVOIDed according to FODMAP categorization**. If you were to see a Yes in the Second Column (Soluble fiber/safe) and a Yes in the FOURTH Column (FODMAP AVOID), you have a clash of approaches, but, you'll notice, this does not occur often, indicating that high FODMAP is generally also not primarily soluble fiber (beans are a stand-out exception). Another interesting point about the FODMAP is that we have a couple categories that are "mixed, depends on how it's prepared", for example, Soy. FODMAP may say that soy in the form of a soybean is high FODMAP/AVOID, but that Soy Sauce is Low FODMAP/SAFE. Using the approach that worked for me, the Common Culprit list suggests that we steer clear of these foods in any form, until we are feeling quite well, consistently, and then reintroduce it, (for example, soy) in its various forms to see if it's an issue. There is nothing wrong with either approach, however I found that eliminating soy altogether, for a period of about three months, was far easier than trying to keep track of which soy was "good" and which was to be avoided.

	The FODMAP diet says these food are safe	These foods are primarily soluble fiber and generally considered safe for IBS	These foods are NOT soluble fiber and may trigger the gastrocolic reflex	The FODMAP diet says these foods are considered High FODMAP and therefore should be avoided
Rice	Yes	Yes		
Banana	Yes	Yes		
Whole Wheat Toast				Yes
Kale	Yes		Yes	
Potatoes, baked	Yes	Yes		
Beans and Legumes		Yes		Yes
Beets, cooked	Yes	Yes		
Carrots, cooked	Yes	Yes		
Cooked oatmeal, plain	Yes	Yes		

Lettuce	Yes		Yes	
Spinach	Yes		Yes	
Eggplant	Yes	Yes		
Blueberries			Yes	YES
Corn		Yes		Yes
Soy	mixed, depends on how its used		Common Culprit, therefore no	Mixed, depends on how it's used
Eggs	Yes		Common culprit, therefore no	
Dairy	mixed, depends on how its used		Common culprit, therefore no	
Yeast	Not listed		Common culprit, therefore no	
Peanuts	Yes		Common culprit, therefore no	
Sugar	Yes		Common culprit, therefore no	

Acknowledgements

Though much of the material for this book is simply a retelling of my journey and sharing of information that I discovered along the way, the book itself materialized with the wonderful support of Christena Smith, my long-time reader and solid friend, and Isabel Detwiler, my number one supporter, encourager and phenomenally snarky editor. I thank you both for, among many things, your unwavering availability as the project evolved.

This 2nd edition would not have come to fruition without the unflagging support, encouragement, and enormously practical advice of Carol Burbank.

I am also immensely grateful for the many individuals who shared your experiences with me, for your honesty and vulnerability. You know who you are.

~Lisa Thorne

ABOUT THE AUTHOR

Lisa Thorne is a holistic wellness coach, author, and photographer. With a background in both the Western medical world and alternative health, Lisa employs her wealth of knowledge, formal education, and life experience to identify the keys to helping others get unstuck and achieve their dreams. After many years traveling and living around the globe, she resides again in her native state of Michigan with her partner, four cats, two dogs, and one snake. Find all her links at: Linktr.ee/LisaThorne.

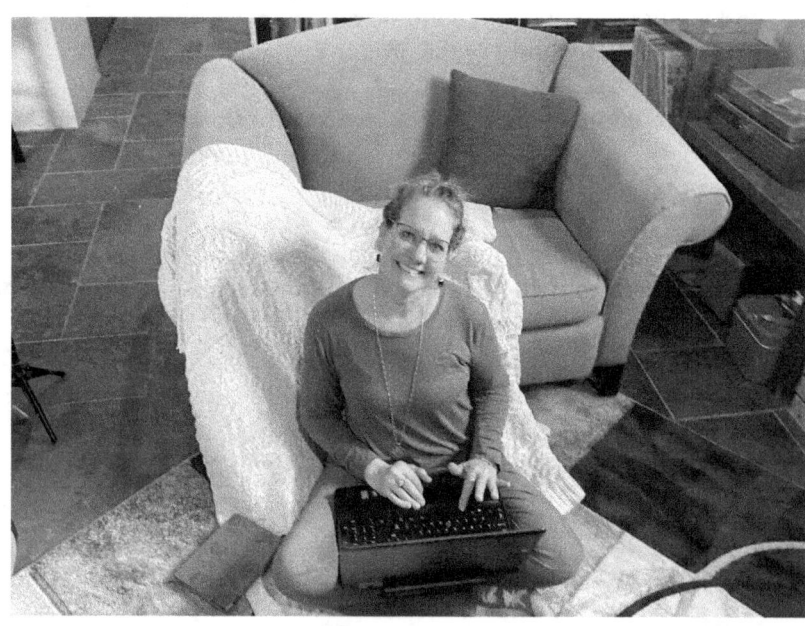

www.ingramcontent.com/pod-product-compliance
Lightning Source LLC
Chambersburg PA
CBHW070721130626
46553CB00005B/2086